Contents

HONEY ORANGE GREEN BEANS

Servings: 4 | Prep: 15m | Cooks: 10m | Total: 45m

NUTRITION FACTS

Calories: 88 | Carbohydrates: 19.6g | Fat: 1.3g | Protein: 1.6g | Cholesterol: 0mg

INGREDIENTS

- 3 tablespoons honey
- 1/2 orange, zested
- 2 cloves garlic, minced
- 1 teaspoon soy sauce
- 1 1/2 teaspoons balsamic vinegar

- 1 dash ground black pepper
- 1 tablespoon water
- 2 cups fresh green beans, trimmed
- 1 teaspoon extra-virgin olive oil
- 1 tomato, diced

DIRECTIONS

1. Stir the honey, orange zest, garlic, soy sauce, balsamic vinegar, pepper, and water together in a bowl. Add the green beans and toss to coat. Allow to soak for 20 minutes, mixing every 5 minutes.
2. Heat the olive oil in a saucepan over low heat; add the green beans to the hot oil and cover the saucepan. Pour the green beans and sauce into the pan and cook, shaking the pan regularly, until the beans are slightly tender, about 5 minutes. Add the tomatoes to the green beans, replace the cover, and continue cooking until the green beans are cooked though yet slightly crispy, about 5 minutes more.

ROASTED CAULIFLOWER "RICE"

Servings: 8 | Prep: 20m | Cooks: 27m | Total: 47m

NUTRITION FACTS

Calories: 59 | Carbohydrates: 7.6g | Fat: 2.8g | Protein: 2.8g | Cholesterol: 0mg

INGREDIENTS

- ooking spray
- 2 heads cauliflower, cut into 1/2-inch pieces

- 1 1/2 tablespoons avocado oil
- 3/4 teaspoon salt, divided

DIRECTIONS

1. Preheat oven to 450 degrees F (230 degrees C). Line 3 baking sheets with aluminum foil and lightly spray with cooking spray.
2. Fill a food processor 1/4 of the way with cauliflower pieces. Pulse 8 to 12 times until cauliflower is the size of rice grains. Transfer to a large bowl. Repeat with remaining cauliflower pieces.
3. Drizzle avocado oil over cauliflower "rice"; toss until well-distributed.
4. Spread 2 1/2 cups of the rice in an even layer on each lined baking sheet.
5. Roast rice until golden, about 16 minutes. Remove from oven, stir well, and spread out again. Return to oven and roast for 6 minutes. Remove from oven, stir well, and spread out again. Continue roasting until browned, about 5 minutes more.
6. Season each sheet of roasted rice with 1/4 teaspoon salt and place in a large container.

ZUCCHINI-TOMATO SAUTE

Servings: 6 | Prep: 20m | Cooks: 25m | Total: 45m

NUTRITION FACTS

Calories: 94 | Carbohydrates: 16.1g | Fat: 2.8g | Protein: 3.2g | Cholesterol: 0mg

INGREDIENTS

- 1 tablespoon vegetable oil
- 1 onion, sliced
- 2 tomatoes, chopped
- 2 pounds zucchini, peeled and cut into 1 inch thick slices
- 1 green bell pepper, chopped
- salt to taste
- ground black pepper to taste
- 1/4 cup uncooked white rice
- 1/2 cup water

DIRECTIONS

1. Heat oil in a saute pan over medium heat. Add onion, and cook and stir for 3 minutes. Add tomatoes, zucchini, and green pepper. Stir. Season to taste with salt and black pepper. Reduce heat, cover, and simmer for 5 minutes.
2. Stir in rice and water. Cover, and cook over low heat for 20 minutes.

THE BEST DRY-ROASTED CHICKPEA RECIPE

Servings: 4 | Prep: 10m | Cooks: 44m | Total: 54m

NUTRITION FACTS

Calories: 105 | Carbohydrates: 16g | Fat: 3.2g | Protein: 3.5g | Cholesterol: 0mg

INGREDIENTS

- 1 (15 ounce) can garbanzo beans, drained and rinsed
- 2 teaspoons olive oil
- 1/4 teaspoon salt, or to taste
- ground black pepper to taste

DIRECTIONS

1. Preheat oven to 425 degrees F (220 degrees C).
2. Spread garbanzo beans in a baking dish and pat dry with a paper towel.
3. Bake in the preheated oven, stirring halfway through, about 22 minutes. Toss with olive oil, salt, and pepper in a large bowl. Return to the baking dish.
4. Continue baking chickpeas, stirring halfway through, until golden and dry on the outside, about 22 minutes more.

STEEL-CUT OATS AND QUINOA BREAKFAST

Servings: 4 | Prep: 5m | Cooks: 20m | Total: 40m

NUTRITION FACTS

Calories: 191 | Carbohydrates: 30.6g | Fat: 4.7g | Protein: 7.6g | Cholesterol: 0mg

INGREDIENTS

- 3 cups water
- 1/2 cup quinoa
- 1/2 cup steel-cut oats
- 2 tablespoons almond meal
- 2 tablespoons flaxseed meal
- 1 tablespoon ground cinnamon

DIRECTIONS

1. Bring water to a boil in a saucepan; add quinoa and oats. Simmer, stirring frequently, until water is absorbed and quinoa is tender, 15 to 20 minutes.
2. Stir almond meal and flaxseed meal into quinoa mixture; pour into a glass container and top with cinnamon. Let cool, about 15 minutes. Transfer to the refrigerator.

MEYER LEMON AVOCADO TOAST

Servings: 2 | Prep: 10m | Cooks: 3m | Total: 13m

NUTRITION FACTS

Calories: 72 | Carbohydrates: 11.8g | Fat: 1.2g | Protein: 3.6g | Cholesterol: 0mg

INGREDIENTS

- 2 slices whole grain bread
- 1/2 avocado
- 2 tablespoons chopped fresh cilantro, or more to taste
- 1 teaspoon Meyer lemon juice, or to taste
- 1/4 teaspoon Meyer lemon zest
- 1 pinch cayenne pepper
- 1 pinch fine sea salt
- 1/4 teaspoon chia seeds

DIRECTIONS

1. Toast bread slices to desired doneness, 3 to 5 minutes.
2. Mash avocado in a bowl; stir in cilantro, Meyer lemon juice, Meyer lemon zest, cayenne pepper, and sea salt. Spread avocado mixture onto toast and top with chia seeds.

SUGAR FREE BLUEBERRY COFFEE CAKE

Servings: 12 | Prep: 15m | Cooks: 40m | Total: 55m

NUTRITION FACTS

Calories: 363 | Carbohydrates: 36.7g | Fat: 21.3g | Protein: 6.7g | Cholesterol: 99mg

INGREDIENTS

- 3/4 cup butter, melted and cooled
- 1 cup milk
- 3 eggs
- 1 teaspoon vanilla extract
- 1 1/2 cups granular sucrolose sweetener (such as Splenda®)
- 2 teaspoons baking powder
- 3 cups all-purpose flour
- 1 3/4 cups fresh or frozen blueberries
- 1 1/2 cups malitol brown sugar substitute
- 3/4 cup flour
- 2 teaspoons ground cinnamon
- 1/2 cup butter, softened

DIRECTIONS

1. Preheat the oven to 350 degrees F (175 degrees C). Grease and flour a 9x13 inch baking pan.
2. In a large bowl, stir together the melted butter, milk, eggs, vanilla and 1 1/2 cups sugar substitute. Combine 3 cups of flour and baking powder; stir into the wet ingredients until just blended. Fold in the blueberries. Spread evenly in the prepared pan.
3. In a small bowl, stir together the brown sugar substitute, 3/4 cup of flour, and cinnamon. Stir in the softened butter with a fork until the mixture is crumbly. Sprinkle over the top of the cake.
4. Bake for 35 to 40 minutes in the preheated oven, until a toothpick inserted into the center of the cake comes out clean. This cake is best served warm.

BLACK BEANS AND RICE

Servings: 10 | Prep: 5m | Cooks: 25m | Total: 30m

NUTRITION FACTS

Calories: 140 | Carbohydrates: 27.1g | Fat: 0.9g | Protein: 6.3g | Cholesterol: 0mg

INGREDIENTS

- 1 teaspoon olive oil
- 1 onion, chopped
- 2 cloves garlic, minced
- 3/4 cup uncooked white rice
- 1 1/2 cups low sodium, low fat vegetable broth
- 1 teaspoon ground cumin
- 1/4 teaspoon cayenne pepper
- 3 1/2 cups canned black beans, drained

DIRECTIONS

1. In a stockpot over medium-high heat, heat the oil. Add the onion and garlic and saute for 4 minutes. Add the rice and saute for 2 minutes.
2. Add the vegetable broth, bring to a boil, cover and lower the heat and cook for 20 minutes. Add the spices and black beans.

CHICKPEA CURRY

Servings: 8 | Prep: 10m | Cooks: 30m | Total: 40m

NUTRITION FACTS

Calories: 135 | Carbohydrates: 20.5g | Fat: 4.5g | Protein: 4.1g | Cholesterol: 0mg

INGREDIENTS

- 2 tablespoons vegetable oil
- 2 onions, minced
- 2 cloves garlic, minced
- 2 teaspoons fresh ginger root, finely chopped
- 6 whole cloves
- 2 (2 inch) sticks cinnamon, crushed
- 1 teaspoon ground cumin
- 1 teaspoon ground coriander
- salt
- 1 teaspoon cayenne pepper
- 1 teaspoon ground turmeric
- 2 (15 ounce) cans garbanzo beans
- 1 cup chopped fresh cilantro

DIRECTIONS

1. Heat oil in a large frying pan over medium heat, and fry onions until tender.
2. Stir in garlic, ginger, cloves, cinnamon, cumin, coriander, salt, cayenne, and turmeric. Cook for 1 minute over medium heat, stirring constantly. Mix in garbanzo beans and their liquid. Continue to cook and stir until all ingredients are well blended and heated through. Remove from heat. Stir in cilantro just before serving, reserving 1 tablespoon for garnish.

SPICY BAKED SWEET POTATO FRIES
Servings: 6 | Prep: 10m | Cooks: 1h | Total: 1h10m

NUTRITION FACTS

Calories: 169 | Carbohydrates: 29.2g | Fat: 4.7g | Protein: 2.1g | Cholesterol: 0mg

INGREDIENTS

- 6 sweet potatoes, cut into French fries
- 2 tablespoons canola oil
- 3 tablespoons taco seasoning mix
- 1/4 teaspoon cayenne pepper

DIRECTIONS

1. Preheat the oven to 425 degrees F (220 degrees C).
2. In a plastic bag, combine the sweet potatoes, canola oil, taco seasoning, and cayenne pepper. Close and shake the bag until the fries are evenly coated. Spread the fries out in a single layer on two large baking sheets.

3. Bake for 30 minutes, or until crispy and brown on one side. Turn the fries over using a spatula, and cook for another 30 minutes, or until they are all crispy on the outside and tender inside. Thinner fries may not take as long.

BAKED SWEET POTATO STICKS
Servings: 6 | Prep: 20m | Cooks: 25m | Total: 45m

NUTRITION FACTS

Calories: 132 | Carbohydrates: 27g | Fat: 1.9g | Protein: 2.6g | Cholesterol: 0mg

INGREDIENTS

- 1 tablespoon olive oil
- 1/2 teaspoon paprika
- 8 sweet potatoes, sliced lengthwise into quarters*

DIRECTIONS

1. Preheat oven to 400 degrees F (200 degrees C). Lightly grease a baking sheet.
2. In a large bowl, mix olive oil and paprika. Add potato sticks, and stir by hand to coat. Place on the prepared baking sheet.
3. Bake 40 minutes in the preheated oven.

WHOLE WHEAT AND HONEY PIZZA DOUGH
Servings: 12 | Prep: 10m | Cooks: 10m | Total: 20m

NUTRITION FACTS

Calories: 83 | Carbohydrates: 17.4g | Fat: 0.6g | Protein: 3.5g | Cholesterol: 0mg

INGREDIENTS

- 1 (.25 ounce) package active dry yeast
- 1 cup warm water
- 2 cups whole wheat flour
- 1/4 cup wheat germ
- 1 teaspoon salt
- 1 tablespoon honey

DIRECTIONS

1. Preheat oven to 350 degrees F (175 degrees C).
2. In a small bowl, dissolve yeast in warm water. Let stand until creamy, about 10 minutes.

3. In a large bowl combine flour, wheat germ and salt. Make a well in the middle and add honey and yeast mixture. Stir well to combine. Cover and set in a warm place to rise for a few minutes.
4. Roll dough on a floured pizza pan and poke a few holes in it with a fork.
5. Bake in preheated oven for 5 to 10 minutes, or until desired crispiness is achieved.

CRANBERRY AND CILANTRO QUINOA SALAD

Servings: 6 | Prep: 10m | Cooks: 20m | Total: 2h30m

NUTRITION FACTS

Calories: 176 | Carbohydrates: 31.6g | Fat: 3.9g | Protein: 5.4g | Cholesterol: 0mg

INGREDIENTS

- 1 1/2 cups water
- cup uncooked quinoa, rinsed
- 1/4 cup red bell pepper, chopped
- 1/4 cup yellow bell pepper, chopped
- 1 small red onion, finely chopped
- 1 1/2 teaspoons curry powder
- 1/4 cup chopped fresh cilantro
- 1 lime, juiced
- 1/4 cup toasted sliced almonds
- 1/2 cup minced carrots
- 1/2 cup dried cranberries
- salt and ground black pepper to taste

DIRECTIONS

1. Pour the water into a saucepan, and cover with a lid. Bring to a boil over high heat, then pour in the quinoa, recover, and continue to simmer over low heat until the water has been absorbed, 15 to 20 minutes. Scrape into a mixing bowl, and chill in the refrigerator until cold.
2. Once cold, stir in the red bell pepper, yellow bell pepper, red onion, curry powder, cilantro, lime juice, sliced almonds, carrots, and cranberries. Season to taste with salt and pepper. Chill before serving.

BROCCOLI SOUP

Servings: 8 | Prep: 15m | Cooks: 25m | Total: 40m

NUTRITION FACTS

Calories: 64 | Carbohydrates: 10.2g | Fat: 2g | Protein: 2.8g | Cholesterol: 0mg

INGREDIENTS

- 1 tablespoon olive oil
- 1 large onion, chopped
- 3 cloves garlic, peeled and chopped
- 2 (10 ounce) packages chopped frozen broccoli, thawed
- 1 potato, peeled and chopped
- 4 cups chicken broth
- 1/4 teaspoon ground nutmeg
- salt and pepper to taste

DIRECTIONS

1. Heat olive oil in a large saucepan, and saute onion and garlic until tender. Mix in broccoli, potato, and chicken broth. Bring to a boil, reduce heat, and simmer 15 minutes, until vegetables are tender.
2. With a hand mixer or in a blender, puree the mixture until smooth. Return to the saucepan, and reheat. Season with nutmeg, salt, and pepper.

GINGERBREAD BISCOTTI

Servings: 48 | Prep: 25m | Cooks: 40m | Total: 1h5m

NUTRITION FACTS

Calories: 70 | Carbohydrates: 12.1g | Fat: 2g | Protein: 1.4g | Cholesterol: 12mg

INGREDIENTS

- 1/3 cup vegetable oil
- 1 cup white sugar
- 3 eggs
- 1/4 cup molasses
- 2 1/4 cups all-purpose flour
- 1 cup whole wheat flour
- 1 tablespoon baking powder
- 1 1/2 tablespoons ground ginger
- 3/4 tablespoon ground cinnamon
- 1/2 tablespoon ground cloves
- 1/4 teaspoon ground nutmeg

DIRECTIONS

1. Preheat the oven to 375 degrees F (190 degrees C). Grease a cookie sheet.
2. In a large bowl, mix together oil, sugar, eggs, and molasses. In another bowl, combine flours, baking powder, ginger, cinnamon, cloves, and nutmeg; mix into egg mixture to form a stiff dough.

3. Divide dough in half, and shape each half into a roll the length of the cookie. Place rolls on cookie sheet, and pat down to flatten the dough to 1/2 inch thickness.
4. Bake in preheated oven for 25 minutes. Remove from oven, and set aside to cool.
5. When cool enough to touch, cut into 1/2 inch thick diagonal slices. Place sliced biscotti on cookie sheet, and bake an additional 5 to 7 minutes on each side, or until toasted and crispy.

MEDITERRANEAN KALE

Servings: 6 | Prep: 15m | Cooks: 10m | Total: 25m

NUTRITION FACTS

Calories: 91 | Carbohydrates: 14.5g | Fat: 3.2g | Protein: 4.6g | Cholesterol: 0mg

INGREDIENTS

- 12 cups chopped kale
- 2 tablespoons lemon juice
- 1 tablespoon olive oil, or as needed
- 1 tablespoon minced garlic
- 1 teaspoon soy sauce
- salt to taste
- ground black pepper to taste

DIRECTIONS

1. Place a steamer insert into a saucepan, and fill with water to just below the bottom of the steamer. Cover, and bring the water to a boil over high heat. Add the kale, recover, and steam until just tender, 7 to 10 minutes depending on thickness.
2. Whisk together the lemon juice, olive oil, garlic, soy sauce, salt, and black pepper in a large bowl. Toss steamed kale into dressing until well coated.

BAKED FRENCH FRIES

Servings: 4 | Prep: 20m | Cooks: 25m | Total: 45m

NUTRITION FACTS

Calories: 145 | Carbohydrates: 28.2g | Fat: 1.6g | Protein: 5.2g | Cholesterol: 4mg

INGREDIENTS

- 3 russet potatoes, sliced into 1/4 inch strips
- cooking spray
- 1/4 cup grated Parmesan cheese
- salt and pepper to taste

* 1 teaspoon dried basil

DIRECTIONS

1. Preheat oven to 400 degrees F (200 degrees C). Lightly grease a medium baking sheet.
2. Arrange potato strips in a single layer on the prepared baking sheet, skin sides down. Spray lightly with cooking spray, and sprinkle with basil, Parmesan cheese, salt and pepper.
3. Bake 25 minutes in the preheated oven, or until golden brown.

SUPERFAST ASPARAGUS

Servings: 3 | Prep: 5m | Cooks: 10m | Total: 15m

NUTRITION FACTS

Calories: 32 | Carbohydrates: 6.3g | Fat: 0.2g | Protein: 3.4g | Cholesterol: 0mg

INGREDIENTS

* 1 pound asparagus
* 1 teaspoon Cajun seasoning

DIRECTIONS

1. Preheat oven to 425 degrees F (220 degrees C).
2. Snap the asparagus at the tender part of the stalk. Arrange spears in one layer on a baking sheet. Spray lightly with nonstick spray; sprinkle with the Cajun seasoning.
3. Bake in the preheated oven until tender, about 10 minutes.

BUTTERNUT SQUASH FRIES

Servings: 4 | Prep: 15m | Cooks: 20m | Total: 35m

NUTRITION FACTS

Calories: 102 | Carbohydrates: 26.5g | Fat: 0.2g | Protein: 2.3g | Cholesterol: 0mg

INGREDIENTS

* 1 (2 pound) butternut squash, halved and seeded
* salt to taste

DIRECTIONS

1. Preheat the oven to 425 degrees F (220 degrees C).
2. Use a sharp knife to carefully cut away the peel from the squash. Cut the squash into sticks like French fries. Arrange squash pieces on a baking sheet and season with salt.
3. Bake for 20 minutes in the preheated oven, turning the fries over halfway through baking. Fries are done when they are starting to brown on the edges and become crispy.

BAKED POTATO

Servings: 1 | Prep: 3m | Cooks: 1h30m | Total: 1h33m

NUTRITION FACTS

Calories: 128 | Carbohydrates: 29.7g | Fat: 0.1g | Protein: 2.7g | Cholesterol: 0mg

INGREDIENTS

- 1 baking potato

DIRECTIONS

1. Preheat oven to 350 degrees F (175 degrees C).
2. Scrub the potato and prick it with a fork to prevent steam from building up and causing the potato to explode in your oven.
3. Bake for 1 1/2 hours.

LENTIL SOUP

Servings: 8 | Prep: 5m | Cooks: 30m | Total: 35m

NUTRITION FACTS

Calories: 156 | Carbohydrates: 27.7g | Fat: 0.7g | Protein: 11.5g | Cholesterol: 0mg

INGREDIENTS

- 2 cups dry lentils
- 2 quarts chicken broth
- 1 onion, diced
- 1/4 cup tomato paste
- 2 cloves garlic, minced
- 1 tablespoon ground cumin

1. In a large saucepan combine lentils, broth, onion, tomato paste, garlic and cumin. Bring to a boil, then reduce heat, cover and simmer until lentils are soft, 30 to 45 minutes. Serve with a squeeze of lemon.

MEXICAN BEAN AND RICE SALAD

Servings: 10 | Prep: 20m | Cooks: 1h | Total: 1h20m

NUTRITION FACTS

Calories: 124 | Carbohydrates: 26g | Fat: 1g | Protein: 4.7g | Cholesterol: 0mg

INGREDIENTS

- 2 cups cooked brown rice
- 1 (15 ounce) can kidney beans, rinsed and drained
- 1 (15 ounce) can black beans, rinsed and drained
- 1 (15.25 ounce) can whole kernel corn, drained
- 1 small onion, diced
- 1 green bell pepper, diced
- 2 jalapeno peppers, seeded and diced
- 1 lime, zested and juiced
- 1/4 cup chopped cilantro leaves
- 1 teaspoon minced garlic
- 1 1/2 teaspoons ground cumin
- salt to taste

DIRECTIONS

1. In a large salad bowl, combine the brown rice, kidney beans, black beans, corn, onion, green pepper, jalapeno peppers, lime zest and juice, cilantro, garlic, and cumin. Lightly toss all ingredients to mix well, and sprinkle with salt to taste.
2. Refrigerate salad for 1 hour, toss again, and serve.

LEMON-ORANGE ORANGE ROUGHY

Servings: 4 | Prep: 15m | Cooks: 5m | Total: 20m

NUTRITION FACTS

Calories: 140 | Carbohydrates: 7.9g | Fat: 4.3g | Protein: 19.1g | Cholesterol: 67mg

INGREDIENTS

- 1 tablespoon olive oil
- 4 (4 ounce) fillets orange roughy
- 1 orange, juiced
- 1 lemon, juiced
- 1/2 teaspoon lemon pepper

DIRECTIONS

1. Heat oil in a large skillet over medium-high heat. Arrange fillets in the skillet, and drizzle with orange juice and lemon juice. Sprinkle with lemon pepper. Cook for 5 minutes, or until fish is easily flaked with a fork.

LEMONY QUINOA

Servings: 6 | Prep: 15m | Cooks: 10m | Total: 25m

NUTRITION FACTS

Calories: 147 | Carbohydrates: 21.4g | Fat: 4.8g | Protein: 5.9g | Cholesterol: 0mg

INGREDIENTS

- 1/4 cup pine nuts
- 1 cup quinoa
- 2 cups water
- sea salt to taste
- 1/4 cup fresh lemon juice
- 2 stalks celery, chopped
- 1/4 red onion, chopped
- 1/4 teaspoon cayenne pepper
- 1/2 teaspoon ground cumin
- 1 bunch fresh parsley, chopped

DIRECTIONS

1. Toast the pine nuts briefly in a dry skillet over medium heat. This will take about 5 minutes, and stir constantly as they will burn easily. Set aside to cool.
2. In a saucepan, combine the quinoa, water and salt. Bring to a boil, then reduce heat to medium and cook until quinoa is tender and water has been absorbed, about 10 minutes. Cool slightly, then fluff with a fork.
3. Transfer the quinoa to a serving bowl and stir in the pine nuts, lemon juice, celery, onion, cayenne pepper, cumin and parsley. Adjust salt and pepper if needed before serving.

FROZEN VEGETABLE STIR-FRY

Servings: 6 | Prep: 5m | Cooks: 5m | Total: 10m

NUTRITION FACTS

Calories: 88 | Carbohydrates: 13.8g | Fat: 2.9g | Protein: 3.5g | Cholesterol: 0mg

INGREDIENTS

- 2 tablespoons soy sauce
- 1 tablespoon brown sugar
- 2 teaspoons garlic powder
- 2 teaspoons peanut butter
- 2 teaspoons olive oil
- 1 (16 ounce) package frozen mixed vegetables

DIRECTIONS

1. Combine soy sauce, brown sugar, garlic powder, and peanut butter in a small bowl.
2. Heat oil in a large skillet over medium heat; cook and stir frozen vegetables until just tender, 5 to 7 minutes. Remove from heat and fold in soy sauce mixture.

GOBI ALOO

Servings: 4 | Prep: 15m | Cooks: 20m | Total: 35m

NUTRITION FACTS

Calories: 135 | Carbohydrates: 23.1g | Fat: 4g | Protein: 4g | Cholesterol: 0mg

INGREDIENTS

- 1 tablespoon vegetable oil
- 1 teaspoon cumin seeds
- 1 teaspoon minced garlic
- 1 teaspoon ginger paste
- 2 medium potatoes, peeled and cubed
- 1/2 teaspoon ground turmeric
- 1/2 teaspoon paprika
- 1 teaspoon ground cumin
- 1/2 teaspoon garam masala
- salt to taste
- 1 pound cauliflower
- 1 teaspoon chopped fresh cilantro

DIRECTIONS

1. Heat the oil in a medium skillet over medium heat. Stir in the cumin seeds, garlic, and ginger paste. Cook about 1 minute until garlic is lightly browned. Add the potatoes. Season with turmeric, paprika, cumin, garam masala, and salt. Cover and continue cooking 5 to 7 minutes stirring occasionally.
2. Mix the cauliflower and cilantro into the saucepan. Reduce heat to low and cover. Stirring occasionally, continue cooking 10 minutes, or until potatoes and cauliflower are tender.

BLACK BEAN SALSA

Servings: 40 | Prep: 15m | Cooks: 8h | Total: 8h15m

NUTRITION FACTS

Calories: 42 | Carbohydrates: 8.3g | Fat: 0.2g | Protein: 2.5g | Cholesterol: 0mg

INGREDIENTS

- 3 (15 ounce) cans black beans, drained and rinsed
- 1 (11 ounce) can Mexican-style corn, drained
- 2 (10 ounce) cans diced tomatoes with green chile peppers, partially drained
- 2 tomatoes, diced
- 2 bunches green onions, chopped
- cilantro leaves, for garnish

DIRECTIONS

1. In a large bowl, mix together black beans, Mexican-style corn, diced tomatoes with green chile peppers, tomatoes and green onion stalks. Garnish with desired amount of cilantro leaves. Chill in the refrigerator at least 8 hours, or overnight, before serving.

EASY LIMA BEANS

Servings: 6 | Prep: 15m | Cooks: 30m | Total: 45m

NUTRITION FACTS

Calories: 84 | Carbohydrates: 15.9g | Fat: 0g | Protein: 4.1g | Cholesterol: 0mg

INGREDIENTS

- cooking spray
- 1/2 medium onion, finely chopped
- 1 1/2 cups chicken broth
- 1 (16 ounce) package frozen baby lima beans

DIRECTIONS

1. Heat a large saucepan over medium heat, and spray with cooking spray. Saute onions until soft and translucent. Pour in chicken broth, and bring to a boil. Add lima beans, and enough water just to cover. Bring to a boil, then reduce heat to low, cover, and simmer for 30 minutes, until beans are tender.

ZUCCHINI WITH CHICKPEA AND MUSHROOM STUFFING

Servings: 8 | Prep: 30m | Cooks: 30m | Total: 1h

NUTRITION FACTS

Calories: 107 | Carbohydrates: 18.4g | Fat: 2.7g | Protein: 4.5g | Cholesterol: 0mg

INGREDIENTS

- 4 zucchini, halved
- 1 tablespoon olive oil
- 1 onion, chopped
- 2 cloves garlic, crushed
- 1/2 (8 ounce) package button mushrooms, sliced
- 1 teaspoon ground coriander
- 1 1/2 teaspoons ground cumin, or to taste
- 1 (15.5 ounce) can chickpeas, rinsed and drained
- 1/2 lemon, juiced
- 2 tablespoons chopped fresh parsley
- sea salt to taste
- ground black pepper to taste

DIRECTIONS

1. Preheat oven to 350 degrees F (175 degrees C). Grease a shallow baking dish.
2. Scoop out the flesh of the zucchini; chop the flesh and set aside. Place the shells in the prepared dish.
3. Heat oil in a large skillet over medium heat. Saute onions for 5 minutes, then add garlic and saute 2 minutes more. Stir in chopped zucchini and mushrooms; saute 5 minutes. Stir in coriander, cumin, chickpeas, lemon juice, parsley, salt and pepper. Spoon mixture into zucchini shells.
4. Bake in preheated oven for 30 to 40 minutes, or until zucchini are tender.

LENTIL RICE AND VEGGIE BAKE

Servings: 6 | Prep: 15m | Cooks: 1h | Total: 1h15m

NUTRITION FACTS

Calories: 187 | Carbohydrates: 35.1g | Fat: 1.5g | Protein: 9.7g | Cholesterol: 0mg

INGREDIENTS

- 1/2 cup uncooked long grain white rice
- 2 1/2 cups water
- 1 cup red lentils
- 1 teaspoon vegetable oil
- 1 small onion, chopped
- 3 cloves garlic, minced
- 1 fresh tomato, chopped
- 1/3 cup chopped celery
- 1/3 cup chopped carrots
- 1/3 cup chopped zucchini
- 1 (8 ounce) can tomato sauce
- 1 teaspoon dried basil
- 1 teaspoon dried oregano
- 1 teaspoon ground cumin
- salt and pepper to taste

DIRECTIONS

1. Place the rice and 1 cup water in a pot, and bring to a boil. Cover, reduce heat to low, and simmer 20 minutes. Place lentils in a pot with the remaining 1 1/2 cups water, and bring to a boil. Cook 15 minutes, or until tender.
2. Preheat oven to 350 degrees F (175 degrees C).
3. Heat the oil in a skillet over medium heat, and stir in the onion and garlic. Mix in tomato, celery, carrots, zucchini, and 1/2 the tomato sauce. Season with 1/2 the basil, 1/2 the oregano, 1/2 the cumin, salt, and pepper. Cook until vegetables are tender.
4. In a casserole dish, mix the rice, lentils, and vegetables. Top with remaining tomato sauce, and sprinkle with remaining basil, oregano, and cumin.
5. Bake 30 minutes in the preheated oven, until bubbly.

QUICK SESAME GREEN BEANS

Servings: 4 | Prep: 10m | Cooks: 5m | Total: 15m

NUTRITION FACTS

Calories: 45 | Carbohydrates: 7.1g | Fat: 1.4g | Protein: 2.3g | Cholesterol: 0mg

INGREDIENTS

- 8 ounces fresh green beans, trimmed
- 4 cloves garlic, minced

- 2 tablespoons low sodium soy sauce
- 1/2 tablespoon miso paste
- 1/2 teaspoon red pepper flakes

- 1 teaspoon grated fresh ginger root
- 1 tablespoon sesame seeds, toasted

DIRECTIONS

1. Place the green beans into a steamer insert and set in a pot over one inch of water. Bring to a boil, cover and steam for 5 minutes. Remove from the heat and transfer beans to a serving bowl.
2. Meanwhile, in a small bowl, stir together the soy sauce, miso paste, red pepper flakes, garlic and ginger. Pour over the green beans and toss to coat. Sprinkle sesame seeds on top.

SAVORY ROASTED ROOT VEGETABLES
Servings: 6 | Prep: 30m | Cooks: 45m | Total: 1h15m

NUTRITION FACTS

Calories: 143 | Carbohydrates: 20.8g | Fat: 4.9g | Protein: 2.8g | Cholesterol: 0mg

INGREDIENTS

- 1 cup diced, raw beet
- 4 carrots, diced
- 1 onion, diced
- 2 cups diced potatoes
- 4 cloves garlic, minced
- 1/4 cup canned garbanzo beans (chickpeas), drained

- 2 tablespoons olive oil
- 1 tablespoon dried thyme leaves
- salt and pepper to taste
- 1/3 cup dry white wine
- 1 cup torn beet greens

DIRECTIONS

1. Preheat an oven to 400 degrees F (200 degrees C).
2. Place the beet, carrot, onion, potatoes, garlic, and garbanzo beans into a 9x13 inch baking dish. Drizzle with the olive oil, then season with thyme, salt, and pepper. Mix well.
3. Bake, uncovered, in the preheated oven for 30 minutes, stirring once midway through baking. Remove the baking dish from the oven, and stir in the wine. Return to the oven, and bake until the wine has mostly evaporated and the vegetables are tender, about 15 minutes more. Stir in the beet greens, allowing them to wilt from the heat of the vegetables. Season to taste with salt and pepper before serving.

CAN'T TELL THEY'RE LOW-FAT BROWNIES

Servings: 12 | Prep: 10m | Cooks: 30m | Total: 40m

NUTRITION FACTS

Calories: 129 | Carbohydrates: 23.9g | Fat: 3.6g | Protein: 2.2g | Cholesterol: 31mg

INGREDIENTS

- 1/2 cup all-purpose flour
- 6 tablespoons unsweetened cocoa powder
- 1 cup white sugar
- 1/8 teaspoon salt
- 2 tablespoons vegetable oil
- 1/2 teaspoon vanilla extract
- 1 (4 ounce) jar pureed prunes baby food
- 2 eggs

DIRECTIONS

1. Preheat oven to 350 degrees F (175 degrees C). Grease an 8x8 inch square pan.
2. In a medium bowl, stir together flour, cocoa, sugar, and salt. Pour in oil, vanilla, prunes, and eggs. Mix until everything is well blended. Spread the batter evenly into the prepared pan.
3. Bake for 30 minutes in the preheated oven, or until top is shiny and a toothpick inserted into the center comes out clean.

SLOW COOKER MEDITERRANEAN STEW

Servings: 10 | Prep: 30m | Cooks: 10h | Total: 10h30m

NUTRITION FACTS

Calories: 122 | Carbohydrates: 30.5g | Fat: 0.5g | Protein: 3.4g | Cholesterol: 0mg

INGREDIENTS

- 1 butternut squash - peeled, seeded, and cubed
- 2 cups cubed eggplant, with peel
- 2 cups cubed zucchini
- 1 (10 ounce) package frozen okra, thawed
- 1 (8 ounce) can tomato sauce
- 1/2 cup vegetable broth
- 1/3 cup raisins
- 1 clove garlic, chopped
- 1/2 teaspoon ground cumin
- 1/2 teaspoon ground turmeric

- 1 cup chopped onion
- 1 ripe tomato, chopped
- 1 carrot, sliced thin
- 1/4 teaspoon crushed red pepper
- 1/4 teaspoon ground cinnamon
- 1/4 teaspoon paprika

DIRECTIONS

1. In a slow cooker, combine butternut squash, eggplant, zucchini, okra, tomato sauce, onion, tomato, carrot, broth, raisins, and garlic. Season with cumin, turmeric, red pepper, cinnamon, and paprika.
2. Cover, and cook on Low for 8 to 10 hours, or until vegetables are tender.

TWICE BAKED SWEET POTATOES WITH RICOTTA CHEESE

Servings: 6 | Prep: 10m | Cooks: 1h30m | Total: 2h

NUTRITION FACTS

Calories: 161 | Carbohydrates: 29.9g | Fat: 2.1g | Protein: 5.5g | Cholesterol: 7mg

INGREDIENTS

- 3 medium sweet potatoes
- 1 teaspoon olive oil
- 2 shallots, finely chopped
- 1/2 cup fat-free ricotta cheese
- 1/4 teaspoon salt
- 1/4 teaspoon ground black pepper
- 1/4 teaspoon ground ginger
- 1 tablespoon brown sugar
- 1/4 cup grated Parmesan cheese
- 2 1/2 tablespoons chopped fresh sage

DIRECTIONS

1. Preheat oven to 400 degrees F (200 degrees C). Pierce potatoes with a fork and bake until soft, about 1 hour. Remove from oven and cool until potatoes can be handled, about 20 minutes.
2. Reduce oven temperature to 350 degrees F (175 degrees C). Grease a large baking sheet.
3. Meanwhile, place olive oil in small skillet over medium heat. Add shallots and cook and stir until softened and beginning to brown, about 10 minutes. Set aside.
4. Cut potatoes in half lengthwise and scoop out pulp, leaving a thin shell. Set shells aside. Place pulp into a blender or food processor and blend until smooth. Add ricotta, salt, pepper, ginger, and sugar to the blender; blend until smooth.
5. Return potato mixture to a bowl; stir in shallots, Parmesan cheese, and sage. Spoon mixture back into potato skins. Place potatoes on prepared baking sheet.
6. Bake until heated through, about 30 minutes.

ROSEMARY ROASTED BUTTERNUT SQUASH

Servings: 6 | Prep: 20m | Cooks: 45m | Total: 1h5m

NUTRITION FACTS

Calories: 136 | Carbohydrates: 24.8g | Fat: 4.7g | Protein: 2.2g | Cholesterol: 0mg

INGREDIENTS

- 1 butternut squash, peeled and cubed
- 2 cloves garlic, minced
- 2 sprigs fresh rosemary, finely chopped
- 2 tablespoons olive oil, or more to taste
- sea salt to taste
- ground black pepper to taste

DIRECTIONS

1. Preheat oven to 400 degrees F (200 degrees C).
2. Mix butternut squash cubes, garlic, rosemary, olive oil, salt, and black pepper until well coated. Spread mixture into a large baking dish.
3. Bake in preheated oven until squash is caramelized and golden brown, 45 to 50 minutes.

COUSCOUS AND CUCUMBER SALAD

Servings: 8 | Prep: 10m | Cooks: 10m | Total: 1h20m

NUTRITION FACTS

Calories: 142 | Carbohydrates: 24.6g | Fat: 3.6g | Protein: 4g | Cholesterol: 0mg

INGREDIENTS

- 10 ounces uncooked couscous
- 2 tablespoons olive oil
- 1/2 cup lemon juice
- 3/4 teaspoon salt
- 1/4 teaspoon ground black pepper
- 1 cucumber, seeded and chopped
- 1/2 cup finely chopped green onions
- 1/2 cup fresh parsley, chopped
- 1/4 cup fresh basil, chopped
- 6 leaves lettuce
- 6 slices lemon
- 1/2 teaspoon lemon pepper

DIRECTIONS

1. In a medium saucepan, bring 1 3/4 cup water to a boil. Stir in couscous; cover. Remove from heat; let stand, covered, 5 minutes. Cool to room temperature.
2. Meanwhile, in a medium bowl combine oil, lemon juice, salt and pepper. Stir in cucumber, green onion, parsley, basil and couscous. Mix well and chill for at least 1 hour.
3. Line a plate with lettuce leaves. Spoon couscous mixture over leaves and garnish with lemon wedges.

HARVESTED CHICKEN STEW

Servings: 10 | Prep: 15m | Cooks: 30m | Total: 45m

NUTRITION FACTS

Calories: 111 | Carbohydrates: 13.1g | Fat: 2.5g | Protein: 10.1g | Cholesterol: 21mg

INGREDIENTS

- 2 cups chopped onion
- 2 cups cubed, cooked boneless chicken breast meat
- 1 cup chopped celery
- 2 cups whole peeled tomatoes, with liquid
- 2 cups sliced carrots
- 5 cups chicken broth
- 1 cup sweet corn
- 1 cup peas
- 1 cup sliced zucchini
- 1/2 teaspoon lemon pepper

DIRECTIONS

1. In a large soup pot combine the onion, chicken, celery, tomatoes with liquid, carrots, broth, corn, peas and zucchini. Stir together and simmer over medium low heat for 1/2 hour, or until vegetables are cooked and tender.

ZESTY ZUCCHINI AND SQUASH

Servings: 6 | Prep: 15m | Cooks: 25m | Total: 40m

NUTRITION FACTS

Calories: 43 | Carbohydrates: 9.7g | Fat: 0.4g | Protein: 1.8g | Cholesterol: 0mg

INGREDIENTS

- 3 medium small yellow squash, cubed
- 1/2 onion, chopped

- 3 small zucchini, cubed
- 1 (10 ounce) can diced tomatoes with green chile peppers
- salt to taste
- garlic powder to taste

DIRECTIONS

1. In a large saucepan, combine squash, zucchini, tomatoes with chiles, onion, salt and garlic powder. Bring to a boil over medium-high heat.
2. Reduce heat to low and cook until tender-crisp.

BANANA OAT BARS

Servings: 18 | Prep: 5m | Cooks: 35m | Total: 45m | Additional: 5m

NUTRITION FACTS

Calories: 72 | Carbohydrates: 16.1g | Fat: 0.5g | Protein: 1.6g | Cholesterol: 0mg

INGREDIENTS

- 1 1/3 cups quick cooking oats
- 1/2 cup white sugar
- 2 teaspoons baking powder
- 1 teaspoon ground cinnamon
- 1/2 teaspoon baking soda
- 1/2 cup raisins
- 1 cup mashed bananas
- 1/4 cup skim milk
- 2 egg whites
- 1 teaspoon vanilla extract

DIRECTIONS

1. Preheat oven to 350 degrees F (175 degrees C).
2. Mix together dry ingredients. In a separate bowl mix together bananas, egg whites, milk and vanilla. Beat all together.
3. Bake in a 9 x 13 inch pan which has been sprayed with non-stick spray for about 35 minutes. Cool and cut into bars. You may sprinkle with cinnamon and sugar, if desired.

GRILLED CORN SALAD

Servings: 6 | Prep: 15m | Cooks: 10m | Total: 1h10m

NUTRITION FACTS

Calories: 103 | Carbohydrates: 19.7g | Fat: 2.8g | Protein: 3.4g | Cholesterol: 0mg

INGREDIENTS

- 6 ears freshly shucked corn
- 1 green pepper, diced
- 2 Roma (plum) tomatoes, diced
- 1/4 cup diced red onion
- 1/2 bunch fresh cilantro, chopped, or more to taste
- 2 teaspoons olive oil, or to taste
- salt and ground black pepper to taste
- 1/2 teaspoon lemon pepper

DIRECTIONS

1. Preheat an outdoor grill for medium heat; lightly oil the grate.
2. Cook the corn on the preheated grill, turning occasionally, until the corn is tender and specks of black appear, about 10 minutes; set aside until just cool enough to handle. Slice the kernels off of the cob and place into a bowl.
3. Combine the warm corn kernels with the green pepper, diced tomato, onion, cilantro, and olive oil. Season with salt and pepper; toss until evenly mixed. Set aside for at least 30 minutes to allow flavors to blend before serving.

MOJITO FRUIT SALAD

Servings: 6 | Prep: 20m | Cooks: 1h | Total: 1h20m

NUTRITION FACTS

Calories: 83 | Carbohydrates: 20.7g | Fat: 0.6g | Protein: 1.3g | Cholesterol: 0mg

INGREDIENTS

- 1 cup cubed seeded watermelon
- 1 cup seedless grapes
- 1 cup cubed cantaloupe
- 1 cup hulled and quartered strawberries
- 1 cup peeled and quartered kiwi
- 1 cup fresh blueberries
- 3 sprigs fresh mint
- 2 teaspoons white sugar
- 3 tablespoons fresh lime juice

DIRECTIONS

1. Mix the watermelon, grapes, cantaloupe, strawberries, and kiwi in a bowl with a tight-fitting lid; top with the blueberries.

2. Stir the mint, sugar, and lime juice together in a bowl, crushing the mint with the back of a spoon while mixing to extract flavors; pour over the fruit mixture. Seal the bowl with lid and refrigerate at least 1 hour.
3. Just before serving, gently flip the sealed bowl several times to coat the fruit with the dressing.

VEGETARIAN BEAN CURRY

Servings: 8 | Prep: 15m | Cooks: 1h10m | Total: 1h25m

NUTRITION FACTS

Calories: 208 | Carbohydrates: 35.9g | Fat: 4.7g | Protein: 8.7g | Cholesterol: 0mg

INGREDIENTS

- 2 tablespoons olive oil
- 1 large white onion, chopped
- 1/2 cup dry lentils
- 2 cloves garlic, minced
- 3 tablespoons curry powder
- 1 teaspoon ground cumin
- 1 pinch cayenne pepper
- 1 (28 ounce) can crushed tomatoes
- 1 (15 ounce) can garbanzo beans, drained and rinsed
- 1 (8 ounce) can kidney beans, drained and rinsed
- 1/2 cup raisins
- salt and pepper to taste

DIRECTIONS

1. Heat the oil in a large pot over medium heat, and cook the onion until tender. Mix in the lentils and garlic, and season with curry powder, cumin, and cayenne pepper. Cook and stir 2 minutes. Stir in the tomatoes, garbanzo beans, kidney beans, and raisins. Season with salt and pepper. Reduce heat to low, and simmer at least 1 hour, stirring occasionally.

PUERTO RICAN TOSTONES

Servings: 2 | Prep: 10m | Cooks: 10m | Total: 20m

NUTRITION FACTS

Calories: 136 | Carbohydrates: 28.5g | Fat: 3.3g | Protein: 1.2g | Cholesterol: 0mg

INGREDIENTS

- 5 tablespoons oil for frying
- 1 green plantain
- 3 cups cold water
- salt to taste

DIRECTIONS

1. Peel the plantain and cut it into 1-inch chunks.
2. Heat the oil in a large skillet. Place the plantains in the oil and fry on both sides,; approximately 3 1/2 minutes per side.
3. Remove the plantains from the pan and flatten the plantains by placing a plate over the fried plantains and pressing down.
4. Dip the plantains in water, then return them to the hot oil and fry 1 minute on each side. Salt to taste and serve immediately.

NO BAKE BUMPY PEANUT BUTTER NUGGETS

Servings: 30 | Prep: 15m | Cooks: 1h | Total: 1h15m

NUTRITION FACTS

Calories: 46 | Carbohydrates: 3.8g | Fat: 2.9g | Protein: 1.9g | Cholesterol: 0mg

INGREDIENTS

- 1/2 cup natural peanut butter
- 1/4 cup nonfat dry milk powder
- 1/4 cup unsweetened flaked coconut
- 1/3 cup rolled oats
- 1/2 teaspoon ground cinnamon
- 1/4 cup wheat germ
- 1/4 cup unsweetened apple juice concentrate, thawed

DIRECTIONS

1. Combine peanut butter, milk powder, and coconut in a large mixing bowl. Stir in oats, ground cinnamon, wheat germ, and apple juice concentrate until thoroughly combined.
2. Shape the mixture into 1 inch balls. Chill thoroughly before serving; store remaining nuggets in the refrigerator.

BAKED BEANS FROM SCRATCH

Servings: 10 | Prep: 10m | Cooks: 8h | Total: 15h30m

NUTRITION FACTS

Calories: 122 | Carbohydrates: 25.9g | Fat: 0.4g | Protein: 4.8g | Cholesterol: 0mg

INGREDIENTS

- 1 cup dried navy beans
- 4 cups water
- 1/4 cup ketchup
- 1/4 cup maple syrup
- 2 tablespoons brown sugar
- 2 tablespoons molasses
- 1 teaspoon Worcestershire sauce
- 1/2 teaspoon salt
- 1/8 teaspoon ground black pepper
- 1/8 teaspoon chili powder
- 1 small onion, chopped

DIRECTIONS

1. Place the navy beans into a large container and cover with several inches of cool water; let stand 8 hours to overnight. Or, bring the beans and water to a boil in a large pot over high heat. Once boiling, turn off the heat, cover, and let stand 1 hour. Drain and rinse before using.
2. Place the beans in a large saucepan with 4 cups of water. Bring to a boil over high heat, then reduce heat to medium-low, cover, and simmer 1 hour.
3. Preheat an oven to 375 degrees F (190 degrees C). Stir the ketchup, maple syrup, brown sugar, molasses, Worcestershire sauce, salt, pepper, and chili powder together in a small bowl; set aside.
4. Once the beans have simmered for 1 hour, drain, and reserve the cooking liquid. Pour the beans into a 1 1/2 quart casserole dish and stir in the chopped onion and the molasses sauce. Stir in enough of the reserved cooking liquid so the sauce covers the beans by 1/4 inch.
5. Cover, and bake in the preheated oven for 10 minutes, then reduce the heat to 200 degrees F (95 degrees C), and cook 6 hours longer. Stir the beans after they have cooked for 3 hours. Once the beans are tender and the sauce has reduced and is sticky, remove from the oven, stir, recover, and allow to stand 15 minutes before serving.

QUINOA CHARD PILAF

Servings: 8 | Prep: 20m | Cooks: 20m | Total: 40m

NUTRITION FACTS

Calories: 224 | Carbohydrates: 36.6g | Fat: 4.7g | Protein: 9.6g | Cholesterol: 0mg

INGREDIENTS

- 1 tablespoon olive oil
- 1 cup canned lentils, rinsed

- 1 onion, diced
- 3 cloves garlic, minced
- 2 cups uncooked quinoa, rinsed
- 8 ounces fresh mushrooms, chopped
- 1 quart vegetable broth
- 1 bunch Swiss chard, stems removed

DIRECTIONS

1. Heat the oil in a large pot over medium heat. Stir in the onion and garlic, and saute 5 minutes, until onion is tender. Mix in quinoa, lentils, and mushrooms. Pour in the broth. Cover, and cook 20 minutes.
2. Remove the pot from heat. Shred chard, and gently mix into the pot. Cover, and allow to sit 5 minutes, or until chard is wilted.

TABBOULEH

Servings: 4 | Prep: 10m | Cooks: 1h | Total: 1h10m

NUTRITION FACTS

Calories: 101 | Carbohydrates: 19.2g | Fat: 3g | Protein: 3.5g | Cholesterol: 0mg

INGREDIENTS

- 1/4 cup bulgur
- 1/2 cup boiling water
- 1 cup chopped parsley
- 1/4 cup chopped fresh mint leaves
- 5 tomatoes, diced
- 1 onion, finely diced
- 2 teaspoons olive oil
- 1 lemon, juiced
- salt to taste

DIRECTIONS

1. Place the bulgur in a small mixing bowl. Add the boiling water, mix and cover with a towel; Let stand for 1 hour. Drain any excess water.
2. Combine the parsley, mint, tomatoes, onion, olive oil, lemon juice and salt. Add the bulgur; mix well and serve.

FRESH TOMATO SALAD

Servings: 7 | Prep: 15m | Cooks: 15m | Total: 30m

NUTRITION FACTS

Calories: 39 | Carbohydrates: 8.6g | Fat: 0.4g | Protein: 1.8g | Cholesterol: 0mg

INGREDIENTS

- 5 tomatoes, diced
- 1 onion, chopped
- 1 cucumber, sliced
- 1 green bell pepper, chopped
- 1/2 cup chopped fresh basil
- 1/2 cup chopped parsley
- 2 tablespoons crushed garlic
- salt and pepper to taste
- 2 tablespoons white wine vinegar

DIRECTIONS

1. In a large bowl, combine the tomato, onion, cucumber, bell pepper, basil, parsley, garlic and vinegar. Toss and add salt and pepper to taste. Chill and serve.

PALEO CHICKEN STEW

Servings: 6 | Prep: 15m | Cooks: 35m | Total: 50m

NUTRITION FACTS

Calories: 145 | Carbohydrates: 20.9g | Fat: 2.5g | Protein: 9.6g | Cholesterol: 21mg

INGREDIENTS

- 2 teaspoons olive oil
- 1 small red onion, chopped
- 2 cloves garlic, minced
- 2 skinless, boneless chicken breast halves, cut into cubes
- 2 sweet potatoes, peeled and chopped
- 1 cup fresh spinach, or to taste
- 1 pinch crushed red pepper, or more to taste
- 1 pinch paprika, or more to taste
- sea salt to taste
- 1/2 cup chicken broth, or more to taste

DIRECTIONS

1. Heat olive oil in a saucepan over medium-high heat. Saute onion and garlic in hot oil until softened, about 5 minutes.
2. Stir chicken, sweet potatoes, spinach, crushed red pepper, paprika, and sea salt with the onion and garlic in the saucepan. Pour as much chicken broth into the saucepan to make the mixture as soup-like or stew-like as you'd like it.
3. Bring the broth to a boil, reduce heat to medium-low, and simmer until the chicken is no longer pink in the middle and the sweet potatoes are tender, about 30 minutes.

EASTER HAM BONE SOUP

Servings: 10 | Prep: 20m | Cooks: 1h55m | Total: 10h15m

NUTRITION FACTS

Calories: 111 | Carbohydrates: 24.8g | Fat: 0.2g | Protein: 3.3g | Cholesterol: 0mg

INGREDIENTS

- 3 quarts water
- 1 ham bone
- 5 potatoes, cut into 1-inch cubes
- 4 cups chopped cabbage
- 2 large stalks celery, chopped
- 5 green onions, chopped, or more to taste
- 1/2 cup water
- 1/3 cup all-purpose flour
- 1 cup light whipping cream

DIRECTIONS

1. Bring 3 quarts water and ham bone to a boil in a large stock pot. Boil until meat from the bone comes off easily, about 1 hour. Remove bone from broth. Allow bone to cool enough to touch; remove as much meat from as possible. Transfer meat to a resealable plastic bag, seal, and refrigerate.
2. Pour broth into a large bowl; cover and refrigerate overnight. Skim and discard any fat from the top of the chilled broth; transfer broth to a large pot.
3. Bring broth to a boil; add potatoes, cabbage, celery, and reserved ham. Continue to simmer until potatoes are tender, about 45 minutes.
4. Whisk 1/2 cup water and flour in a bowl; whisk into potato-ham soup until thickened. Add light cream; stir.

CHICKEN PASTA

Servings: 8 | Prep: 30m | Cooks: 15m | Total: 45m

NUTRITION FACTS

Calories: 185 | Carbohydrates: 26.1g | Fat: 1.8g | Protein: 15.7g | Cholesterol: 27mg

INGREDIENTS

- 3 cups mostaccioli
- 3 skinless, boneless chicken breast halves
- 1/4 onion, chopped
- 3 fresh mushrooms, sliced
- 2 tablespoons Italian seasoning
- 1 (14.5 ounce) can diced tomatoes
- salt and pepper to taste
- 2 tablespoons grated Parmesan cheese

DIRECTIONS

1. Bring a large pot of lightly salted water to a boil. Add pasta and cook for 8 to 10 minutes or until al dente; drain and reserve.
2. Meanwhile, in a large lightly greased skillet over medium heat, cook chicken for about 15 minutes and remove from pan; cool and dice.
3. In a large skillet over medium heat, combine onion, mushrooms, Italian seasoning, tomatoes with juice, salt and pepper; cook until onions are translucent. Remove from heat and add chicken and pasta. Sprinkle Parmesan cheese on top; serve.

BUTTERNUT SQUASH CAJUN FRIES

Servings: 6 | Prep: 20m | Cooks: 25m | Total: 45m

NUTRITION FACTS

Calories: 52 | Carbohydrates: 13.5g | Fat: 0.1g | Protein: 1.2g | Cholesterol: 0mg

INGREDIENTS

- cooking spray
- 1 pound butternut squash - peeled, seeded, and cut into thick French fries
- 1 pinch salt to taste
- 1/4 teaspoon ground black pepper, or to taste
- 1/2 teaspoon Cajun seasoning, or to taste

DIRECTIONS

1. Preheat oven to 450 degrees F (230 degrees C). Spray a baking sheet with cooking spray.
2. Blot any moisture from the butternut squash fries with paper towels, and place on the prepared baking sheet. Sprinkle with salt, black pepper, and Cajun seasoning.
3. Bake in the preheated oven until lightly browned and tender, 15 to 20 minutes, turning once.

CABBAGE ON THE GRILL

Servings: 8 | Prep: 15m | Cooks: 40m | Total: 55m

NUTRITION FACTS

Calories: 41 | Carbohydrates: 9.4g | Fat: 0.2g | Protein: 2.1g | Cholesterol: 0mg

INGREDIENTS

- 1 large head cabbage
- salt and pepper to taste
- 1 1/2 teaspoons garlic powder, or to taste

DIRECTIONS

1. Preheat grill for medium heat.
2. Cut the cabbage into 8 wedges, and remove the core. Place all the wedges on a piece of aluminum foil large enough to wrap the cabbage. Season to taste with garlic powder, salt, and pepper. Seal cabbage in the foil.
3. Grill for 30 to 40 minutes on the preheated grill, until tender.

COUSCOUS WITH MUSHROOMS AND SUN-DRIED TOMATOES

Servings: 4 | Prep: 30m | Cooks: 15m | Total: 45m

NUTRITION FACTS

Calories: 178 | Carbohydrates: 36.1g | Fat: 2g | Protein: 7.5g | Cholesterol: 0mg

INGREDIENTS

- 1 cup dehydrated sun-dried tomatoes
- 1 1/2 cups water
- 1/2 (10 ounce) package couscous
- 1/3 cup fresh basil leaves
- 1/4 cup fresh cilantro, chopped
- 1/2 lemon, juiced

- 1 teaspoon olive oil
- 3 cloves garlic, pressed
- 1 bunch green onions, chopped
- salt and pepper to taste
- 4 ounces portobello mushroom caps, sliced

DIRECTIONS

1. Place the sun-dried tomatoes in a bowl with 1 cup water. Soak 30 minutes, until rehydrated. Drain, reserving water, and chop.
2. In a medium saucepan, combine the reserved sun-dried tomato water with enough water to yield 1 1/2 cups. Bring to a boil. Stir in the couscous. Cover, remove from heat, and allow to sit 5 minutes, until liquid has been absorbed. Gently fluff with a fork.
3. Heat the olive oil in a skillet. Stir in the sun-dried tomatoes, garlic, and green onions. Cook and stir about 5 minutes, until the green onions are tender. Mix in the basil, cilantro, and lemon juice. Season with salt and pepper. Mix in the mushrooms, and continue cooking 3 to 5 minutes. Toss with the cooked couscous to serve.

LENTIL CHILI

Servings: 12 | Prep: 25m | Cooks: 1h | Total: 1h25m

NUTRITION FACTS

Calories: 189 | Carbohydrates: 32.6g | Fat: 3.1g | Protein: 10.9g | Cholesterol: 3mg

INGREDIENTS

- 1 tablespoon olive oil
- 1 tablespoon butter
- 4 cups chopped onion
- 1 bulb garlic cloves, chopped
- 1 (16 ounce) package dry lentils
- 1 (6 ounce) can tomato paste
- 1 (14.5 ounce) can crushed tomatoes
- 2 quarts water
- 2 tablespoons chili powder
- 1 tablespoon cumin
- 1 dash paprika
- salt to taste
- black pepper to taste
- 2 cups sliced carrots
- 2 cups sliced celery

DIRECTIONS

1. Heat the olive oil and melt the butter in a large pot over low heat. Stir in onion and garlic, and cook until tender. Mix in lentils, tomato paste, and crushed tomatoes. Pour in the water. Season chili with chili powder, cumin, paprika, salt, and pepper. Bring to a boil. Reduce heat to low, cover, and simmer 30 minutes, stirring occasionally.
2. Mix carrots and celery into the chili. Continue cooking 20 minutes over low heat, until lentils, carrots, and celery are tender.

MARINATED BEET SALAD

Servings: 4 | Prep: 10m | Cooks: 10m | Total: 4h20m

NUTRITION FACTS

Calories: 89 | Carbohydrates: 21.7g | Fat: 0.2g | Protein: 1.2g | Cholesterol: 0mg

INGREDIENTS

- 1 (16 ounce) can whole beets
- 1/4 cup white wine vinegar
- 1/4 cup white sugar
- 1/4 cup diced red onion
- 1 teaspoon prepared mustard

DIRECTIONS

1. Drain beets, reserving 1/4 cup liquid, and slice into 1/4 to 1/2 inch slivers. Add onions and toss.
2. In a saucepan over medium heat, cook the sugar, mustard and reserved 1/4 cup liquid until dissolved. Add vinegar and bring to boil; remove from heat and allow to cool.
3. Pour over the beet slices and onions, toss and refrigerate for 4 to 6 hours. Remove from refrigerator and serve at room temperature.

CURRIED CUMIN POTATOES

Servings: 8 | Prep: 15m | Cooks: 20m | Total: 35m

NUTRITION FACTS

Calories: 128 | Carbohydrates: 21.4g | Fat: 4g | Protein: 2.7g | Cholesterol: 0mg

INGREDIENTS

- 2 pounds new potatoes, cut into 1/4 inch thick pieces
- 2 teaspoons curry powder
- 2 tablespoons olive oil
- 2 teaspoons coarse sea salt
- 2 tablespoons cumin seed
- 1 teaspoon ground black pepper

- 2 teaspoons ground turmeric
- 3 tablespoons chopped fresh cilantro

DIRECTIONS

1. Place whole potatoes into a saucepan with water to cover. Bring to a boil, and cook until just tender. Drain, and cut potatoes into quarters. Set aside to keep warm.
2. Heat oil in a large saute pan over medium-high heat. Saute the cumin, turmeric, and curry powder for 1 minute. Add potatoes, and saute until toasted. Toss potatoes with sea salt, pepper and fresh cilantro, and serve hot.

TORTILLA SOUP

Servings: 6 | Prep: 20m | Cooks: 50m | Total: 1h10m

NUTRITION FACTS

Calories: 148 | Carbohydrates: 16.5g | Fat: 2.8g | Protein: 14.8g | Cholesterol: 35mg

INGREDIENTS

- 9 cups chicken broth
- 6 cloves roasted garlic
- 1/2 cup chopped tomatoes
- 1/2 yellow onion, chopped
- 2 fresh jalapeno peppers, sliced into rings
- 1 teaspoon dried oregano
- 1/2 yellow onion, sliced
- 2 cups shredded, cooked chicken meat
- 1 lime, juiced
- 6 (6 inch) corn tortillas, cut into strips and toasted for garnish

DIRECTIONS

1. In heavy pot, bring the broth to a boil. Add garlic, tomatoes, chopped onion, jalapeno, and oregano to the stocks. Simmer uncovered for 30 minutes.
2. Broil the sliced onions until soft and a little brown. Add broiled onions, chicken, lime juice to soup, and simmer till chicken is heated.
3. Place toasted tortilla strips in each bowl and pour soup over strips.

PUMPKIN PROTEIN COOKIES

Servings: 14 | Prep: 15m | Cooks: 5m | Total: 20m

NUTRITION FACTS

Calories: 85 | Carbohydrates: 13.1g | Fat: 2.2g | Protein: 4.2g | Cholesterol: 0mg

INGREDIENTS

- 3/4 cup SPLENDA® Granular
- 1 cup rolled oats
- 1 cup whole wheat flour
- 1/2 cup soy flour
- 1 3/4 teaspoons baking soda
- 1/2 teaspoon baking powder
- 1/2 teaspoon salt
- 2 teaspoons ground cinnamon
- 1 teaspoon ground nutmeg
- 1/2 cup pumpkin puree
- 1 tablespoon canola oil
- 2 teaspoons water
- 2 egg whites
- 1 teaspoon molasses
- 1 tablespoon flax seeds (optional)

DIRECTIONS

1. Preheat oven to 350 degrees F (175 degrees C).
2. In a large bowl, whisk together Splenda®, oats, wheat flour, soy flour, baking soda, baking powder, salt, cinnamon, and nutmeg. Stir in pumpkin, canola oil, water, egg whites, and molasses. Stir in flax seeds, if desired. Roll into 14 large balls, and flatten on a baking sheet.
3. Bake for 5 minutes in preheated oven. DO NOT OVERBAKE: the cookies will come out really dry if overbaked.

COLLARD GREENS AND BEANS

Servings: 4 | Prep: 10m | Cooks: 2h25m | Total: 2h35m

NUTRITION FACTS

Calories: 163 | Carbohydrates: 24.8g | Fat: 3.5g | Protein: 8.3g | Cholesterol: 7mg

INGREDIENTS

- 3 slices bacon, coarsely chopped
- 1 red onion, thinly sliced
- 1 tablespoon brown sugar
- 2 teaspoons cider vinegar

- 2 tablespoons minced garlic, or to taste
- 5 cups collard greens, stems and center ribs discarded and leaves chopped
- 3/4 cup water, or as needed
- 1 teaspoon crushed red pepper flakes, or to taste
- salt and black pepper to taste
- 1 (15 ounce) can cannellini beans, drained and rinsed

DIRECTIONS

1. Place the bacon in a large, deep pan with a lid, and cook over medium-high heat, stirring occasionally, until evenly browned, about 10 minutes. Remove the bacon pieces from the pan, and set aside.
2. Reduce the heat to medium-low, and stir the sliced onion into the hot bacon fat. Cook and stir the onion until it begins to brown, scraping the bits off the bottom of the pan, about 8 minutes. Add the garlic, and cook and stir 4 more minutes. Return the bacon to the pan, stir in the collard greens, and toss gently until the greens are wilted, about 3 minutes.
3. Pour in the water to almost cover the collard greens, and stir in the brown sugar, vinegar, crushed red pepper, and salt and pepper. Bring to a boil, cover, reduce heat to low, and simmer the collard greens until very tender, 1 to 2 hours.
4. About 1/2 hour before serving, stir the cannellini beans into the collard greens, and return to a simmer.

BANANA BREAKFAST COOKIES

Servings: 12 | Prep: 10m | Cooks: 20m | Total: 45m | Additional: 15m

NUTRITION FACTS

Calories: 123 | Carbohydrates: 27.4g | Fat: 1.1g | Protein: 2.9g | Cholesterol: 0mg

INGREDIENTS

- 3 very ripe bananas
- 2 cups rolled oats
- 1 cup raisins
- 1/3 cup plain yogurt
- 1 teaspoon ground cinnamon

DIRECTIONS

1. Preheat the oven to 350 degrees F (175 degrees C). Line cookie sheets with parchment paper.
2. Mash bananas in a large bowl. Add oats, raisins, yogurt, and cinnamon. Mix well and allow to sit for 15 minutes.
3. Drop spoonfuls of dough 2 inches apart onto the prepared cookie sheets.
4. Bake in the preheated oven until lightly browned, about 20 minutes.

TRAIL MIX COOKIES

Servings: 36 | Prep: 20m | Cooks: 10m | Total: 30m

NUTRITION FACTS

Calories: 77 | Carbohydrates: 14.1g | Fat: 2g | Protein: 1.4g | Cholesterol: 0mg

INGREDIENTS

- 1/2 cup applesauce
- 1/2 cup white sugar
- 1/2 cup brown sugar
- 1 1/2 teaspoons vanilla extract
- 2 egg whites
- 1 1/4 cups all-purpose flour
- 1 teaspoon baking soda
- 1/2 teaspoon salt
- 3/4 teaspoon ground cinnamon
- 1 1/4 cups quick cooking oats
- 1/2 cup semisweet chocolate chips
- 1/2 cup chopped walnuts
- 1/3 cup dried cranberries

DIRECTIONS

1. Preheat oven to 350 degrees F (175 degrees C). Grease 2 baking sheets.
2. Beat applesauce, white sugar, brown sugar, and vanilla in a large bowl. In another bowl, use an electric mixer to beat egg whites until they are frothy and begin to firm up. Fold egg whites into applesauce mixture. Combine the flour, baking soda, salt, and cinnamon. Fold into the egg mixture. Stir in the oats, chocolate chips, walnuts, and cranberries. Drop by heaping teaspoons on prepared baking sheets.
3. Bake cookies in preheated oven until set and lightly browned, about 10 minutes. Remove immediately to wire racks to cool.

SPLIT PEA SOUP WITHOUT PORK

Servings: 10 | Prep: 15m | Cooks: 2h | Total: 2h15m

NUTRITION FACTS

Calories: 65 | Carbohydrates: 11.2g | Fat: 0.3g | Protein: 4.8g | Cholesterol: 0mg

INGREDIENTS

- 1 pound dried split peas
- 2 (14.5 ounce) cans low-fat, low sodium chicken broth

- 1 stalk celery, diced
- 2 large carrots, peeled and diced
- 3 cups water
- salt and pepper to taste

DIRECTIONS

1. Rinse and pick through peas. Place them in a large pot with the celery, carrots, broth and water. Bring to a boil, then reduce heat, cover and simmer until peas have fallen apart, 1 to 2 hours. Season with salt and pepper before serving.

SLOW COOKER PUMPKIN STEEL CUT OATS
Servings: 8 | Prep: 5m | Cooks: 6h | Total: 6h5m

NUTRITION FACTS

Calories: 195 | Carbohydrates: 38.2g | Fat: 2.9g | Protein: 5.9g | Cholesterol: 0mg

INGREDIENTS

- cooking spray (such as Pam®)
- 6 cups water
- 1 (15 ounce) can pumpkin puree
- 1 1/2 cups steel-cut oats
- 1 cup brown sugar replacement (such as Splenda® Brown Sugar Blend)
- 2 tablespoons ground cinnamon
- 1 tablespoon pumpkin pie spice

DIRECTIONS

1. Prepare the crock of your slow cooker with cooking spray.
2. Stir water, pumpkin puree, oats, brown sugar replacement, cinnamon, and pumpkin pie spice together in the prepared slow cooker.
3. Cook on Low for 6 hours. Stir before serving.

QUINOA PORRIDGE
Servings: 3 | Prep: 5m | Cooks: 30m | Total: 35m

NUTRITION FACTS

Calories: 173 | Carbohydrates: 31.3g | Fat: 3g | Protein: 4.3g | Cholesterol: 0mg

INGREDIENTS

- 1/2 cup quinoa
- 1/4 teaspoon ground cinnamon
- 1 1/2 cups almond milk
- 1/2 cup water
- 2 tablespoons brown sugar
- 1 teaspoon vanilla extract (optional)
- 1 pinch salt

DIRECTIONS

1. Heat a saucepan over medium heat and measure in the quinoa. Season with cinnamon and cook until toasted, stirring frequently, about 3 minutes. Pour in the almond milk, water and vanilla and stir in the brown sugar and salt. Bring to a boil, then cook over low heat until the porridge is thick and grains are tender, about 25 minutes. Add more water if needed if the liquid has dried up before it finishes cooking. Stir occasionally, especially at the end, to prevent burning.

BANANA OAT ENERGY BARS

Servings: 12 | Prep: 15m | Cooks: 20m | Total: 35m

NUTRITION FACTS

Calories: 124 | Carbohydrates: 20g | Fat: 4g | Protein: 3.6g | Cholesterol: 0mg

INGREDIENTS

- 2 cups rolled oats
- 2 bananas, mashed
- 2 carrots, grated
- 1 apple, grated
- 1 cup unsweetened applesauce
- 1/2 cup chopped peanuts

DIRECTIONS

1. Preheat oven to 350 degrees F (175 degrees C). Grease a 9x13-inch baking dish.
2. Mix oats, bananas, carrots, apple, applesauce, and peanuts together in a bowl; spread into the prepared baking dish.
3. Bake in the preheated oven until golden brown, about 20 minutes.

RAW HUMMUS

Servings: 20 | Prep: 15m | Cooks: 2m | Total: 3d17m

NUTRITION FACTS

Calories: 67 | Carbohydrates: 10.8g | Fat: 1.8g | Protein: 3.3g | Cholesterol: 0mg

INGREDIENTS

- 1 1/2 cups dry garbanzo beans
- 2 tablespoons tahini
- 1 teaspoon sea salt
- 2 lemons, juiced
- 4 cloves garlic, crushed or to taste
- 1 cup filtered or spring water
- 1 pinch paprika

DIRECTIONS

1. Soak the beans for 24 hours. Drain, and let sit for 2 to 3 days, until the bean's sprouts are about 1/2 inch long. Rinse the beans once or twice a day.
2. Bring a large pot of water to a boil. Remove from heat, and let stand for 1 minute. Place the sprouted beans in the hot water, and let sit for 1 minute. Drain. If you do not do this step, the hummus will be awful.
3. Place the sprouted beans into the container of a large food processor. Add the tahini, sea salt, lemon juice, and garlic. Process until smooth, adding water if necessary. It will take 3 to 5 minutes to blend. Let sit in the food processor for 5 minutes to allow the beans to absorb as much of the water as possible. If too thick, add more water, and blend again. Taste and adjust seasonings if needed. Spoon into a serving dish, and garnish with paprika.

SUPER EASY SLOW COOKER CHICKEN ENCHILADA MEAT

Servings: 10 | Prep: 15m | Cooks: 8h | Total: 8h15m

Calories: 93 | Carbohydrates: 8.8g | Fat: 1.8g | Protein: 10.4g | Cholesterol: 23mg

INGREDIENTS

- 2 cups chicken broth
- 1 (14.5 ounce) can diced tomatoes
- 1/3 cup chili powder
- 1/2 cup all-purpose flour
- 1 clove garlic

- 2 teaspoons ground cumin
- 1 teaspoon oregano
- 1 teaspoon salt, or to taste
- 1 pinch cayenne pepper, or more to taste (optional)
- 4 skinless, boneless chicken breast halves

DIRECTIONS

1. Blend chicken broth, tomatoes, chili powder, flour, garlic, cumin, oregano, salt, and cayenne pepper in a blender until smooth.
2. Put chicken breast in bottom of a slow cooker; pour blended enchilada sauce over the chicken.
3. Cook on Low 8 to 9 hours (or 4 to 6 hours on High). Shred the chicken with 2 large forks and stir into the sauce.

ITALIAN STEWED TOMATOES

Servings: 9 | Prep: 30m | Cooks: 10m | Total: 40m

NUTRITION FACTS

Calories: 100 | Carbohydrates: 22.2g | Fat: 1g | Protein: 4.6g | Cholesterol: 0mg

INGREDIENTS

- 24 large tomatoes - peeled, seeded and chopped
- 1 cup chopped celery
- 1/2 cup chopped onion

- 1/4 cup chopped green bell pepper
- 2 teaspoons dried basil
- 1 tablespoon white sugar

DIRECTIONS

1. In a large saucepan over medium heat, combine tomatoes, celery, onion, bell pepper, basil and sugar. Cover and cook for 10 minutes, stirring occasionally to prevent sticking.

CURRIED LENTILS

Servings: 2 | Prep: 20m | Cooks: 20m | Total: 40m

NUTRITION FACTS

Calories: 145 | Carbohydrates: 25.2g | Fat: 0.5g | Protein: 10.8g | Cholesterol: 0mg

INGREDIENTS

- 1/2 cup dried lentils
- 1 cup water
- 3/4 cup canned cream of coconut
- 1 tablespoon curry paste
- salt to taste

DIRECTIONS

1. Rinse lentils and place in a saucepan with the water. Bring to a boil, then cover, and simmer over low heat for 15 minutes. Stir in the curry paste, coconut cream and season with salt to taste. Return to a simmer, and cook for an additional 10 to 15 minutes, until tender.

ALL-STAR VEGGIE BURGER

Servings: 8 | Prep: 20m | Cooks: 10m | Total: 30m

NUTRITION FACTS

Calories: 161 | Carbohydrates: 23.8g | Fat: 4.7g | Protein: 8.3g | Cholesterol: 0mg

INGREDIENTS

- 1 (15.5 ounce) can garbanzo beans, drained and mashed
- 8 fresh basil leaves, chopped
- 1/4 cup oat bran
- 1/4 cup quick cooking oats
- 1 cup cooked brown rice
- 1 (14 ounce) package firm tofu
- 5 tablespoons Korean barbeque sauce
- 1/2 teaspoon salt
- 1/2 teaspoon ground black pepper
- 3/4 teaspoon garlic powder
- 3/4 teaspoon dried sage
- 2 teaspoons vegetable oil

DIRECTIONS

1. In a large bowl, stir together the mashed garbanzo beans and basil. Mix in the oat bran, quick oats, and rice; the mixture should seem a little dry.
2. In a separate bowl, mash the tofu with your hands, trying to squeeze out as much of the water as possible. Drain of the water, and repeat the process until there is hardly any water worth pouring off. It is not necessary to remove all of the water. Pour the barbeque sauce over the tofu, and stir to coat.
3. Stir the tofu into the garbanzo beans and oats. Season with salt, pepper, garlic powder, and sage; mix until well blended.
4. Heat the oil in a large skillet over medium-high heat. Form patties out of the bean mixture, and fry them in hot oil for about 5 minutes per side. Serve as you would burgers.

CHILLED CANTALOUPE SOUP

Servings: 6 | Prep: 20m | Cooks: 1h | Total: 1h20m

NUTRITION FACTS

Calories: 69 | Carbohydrates: 16.4g | Fat: 0.3g | Protein: 1.4g | Cholesterol: 0mg

INGREDIENTS

- 1 cantaloupe - peeled, seeded and cubed
- 2 cups orange juice
- 1 tablespoon fresh lime juice
- 1/4 teaspoon ground cinnamon

DIRECTIONS

1. Peel, seed, and cube the cantaloupe.
2. Place cantaloupe and 1/2 cup orange juice in a blender or food processor; cover, and process until smooth. Transfer to large bowl. Stir in lime juice, cinnamon, and remaining orange juice. Cover, and refrigerate for at least one hour. Garnish with mint if desired.

WHITE BEANS AND PEPPERS

Servings: 4 | Prep: 10m | Cooks: 15m | Total: 25m

NUTRITION FACTS

Calories: 150 | Carbohydrates: 26.6g | Fat: 1.8g | Protein: 8.5g | Cholesterol: 0mg

INGREDIENTS

- 1 teaspoon olive oil
- 1/4 large onion, chopped
- 1 pinch dried oregano
- ground cayenne pepper to taste

- 1 yellow gypsy (bull horn) sweet pepper, chopped
- 1 (15 ounce) can great Northern beans, drained
- salt to taste
- ground black pepper to taste

DIRECTIONS

1. Heat the oil in a skillet over medium heat. Stir in onion and sweet pepper, and cook until tender. Mix in beans. Season with oregano, cayenne pepper, salt, and black pepper. Continue cooking, stirring occasionally, until beans are heated through.

PARSLEY POTATOES

Servings: 6 | Prep: 15m | Cooks: 15m | Total: 30m

NUTRITION FACTS

Calories: 134 | Carbohydrates: 23.5g | Fat: 2.9g | Protein: 4.3g | Cholesterol: <1mg

INGREDIENTS

- 1 1/2 pounds new red potatoes
- 1 tablespoon vegetable oil
- 1 onion, chopped
- 1 clove garlic, crushed
- 1 cup chicken broth
- 1 cup chopped fresh parsley
- 1/2 teaspoon ground black pepper
- 1/2 teaspoon lemon pepper

DIRECTIONS

1. Peel a strip of skin from around the center of each potato, place the potatoes in cold water. Set aside.
2. Heat oil in a large skillet over medium high heat. Saute onion and garlic for 5 minutes or until tender. Pour in broth and 3/4 cup of the parsley; mix well. Bring to a boil.
3. Place the potatoes into a large pot full of salted water. Bring the water to a boil; then reduce heat. Simmer covered, for 10 minutes or until the potatoes are tender.
4. Remove potatoes with a slotted spoon to a serving bowl. Sprinkle the black pepper into the skillet and stir.. Pour the peppered sauce over potatoes and sprinkle with remaining parsley.

PUMPKIN PIE FOR DIETERS

Servings: 6 | Prep: 10m | Cooks: 1h | Total: 1h10m | Additional: 1h

NUTRITION FACTS

Calories: 110 | Carbohydrates: 23g | Fat: 0.3g | Protein: 1.5g | Cholesterol: 0mg

INGREDIENTS

- 1 (15 ounce) can pumpkin puree
- 1/2 cup skim milk
- 1 (1 ounce) package instant sugar-free vanilla pudding mix
- 1 teaspoon pumpkin pie spice
- 1 (8 ounce) container fat free frozen whipped topping
- 1/2 teaspoon lemon pepper

DIRECTIONS

1. In a medium bowl, mix together the pumpkin, milk, and instant pudding mix. Stir in the pumpkin pie spice, and fold in half of the whipped topping.
2. Pour into an 8-inch pie plate, and spread remaining whipped topping over the top. Chill for 1 hour, or until set.

SLOW COOKER CIDER APPLESAUCE

Servings: 16 | Prep: 10m | Cooks: 4h | Total: 4h10m

NUTRITION FACTS

Calories: 76 | Carbohydrates: 20.2g | Fat: 0.3g | Protein: 0.4g | Cholesterol: 0mg

INGREDIENTS

- pounds apples - peeled, cored, and thinly sliced
- 1 1/2 tablespoons ground cinnamon
- 1/2 teaspoon ground cloves
- 1/4 teaspoon ground nutmeg

DIRECTIONS

1. Layer apples into a slow cooker. Sprinkle cinnamon, cloves, and nutmeg over the apples.
2. Cook on High until apples are soft, 4 to 5 hours. Whisk apples vigorously for a chunkier-style applesauce. Puree with an immersion blender for a smoother applesauce.

SHREDDED POTATO SALMON CAKES

Servings: 12 | Prep: 25m | Cooks: 6m | Total: 31m

NUTRITION FACTS

Calories: 139 | Carbohydrates: 15.9g | Fat: 4.6g | Protein: 8.7g | Cholesterol: 42mg

INGREDIENTS

- 3 medium potatoes, peeled and shredded
- 2 eggs
- salt and pepper to taste
- 1 teaspoon Italian seasoning
- 1/2 pound cooked flaked salmon
- 3 green onions, chopped
- 2 tablespoons capers, drained
- 1 red bell pepper, seeded and chopped
- 3/4 cup chopped canned banana peppers
- 3/4 cup sliced fresh mushrooms
- 3/4 cup dry bread crumbs
- 1 cup oil for frying, or as needed

DIRECTIONS

1. Squeeze as much liquid from the potatoes as you can, and place in a large bowl. Beat the eggs with salt, pepper, and Italian seasoning, and mix with the potatoes. Mix in salmon, green onions, capers, red bell pepper, banana peppers, mushrooms and bread crumbs. Form into about 12 patties about 3/4 inch thick.
2. Heat 1/4 inch of oil in a large heavy skillet over medium-high heat. Fry the patties for about 3 minutes per side, or until golden brown. Drain on paper towels quickly before serving. Try to fry all the patties at one time, otherwise the mixture becomes stiff.

EASY SPICED BROWN RICE WITH CORN
Servings: 6 | Prep: 5m | Cooks: 1h | Total: 1h5m

NUTRITION FACTS

Calories: 133 | Carbohydrates: 24.4g | Fat: 3.2g | Protein: 2.7g | Cholesterol: 0mg

INGREDIENTS

- 2 cups water
- 1 cup brown rice
- 1 tablespoon olive oil
- 1/2 teaspoon salt
- 1 cup frozen corn kernels
- 1/2 teaspoon dried cilantro
- 1/2 teaspoon cumin seed

DIRECTIONS

1. In a saucepan, mix the water, rice, olive oil, and salt, and bring to a boil. Mix in the corn, cilantro, and cumin. Reduce heat, cover, and simmer 45 to 60 minutes, until the liquid has been absorbed.

BLACK BEAN AND RICE SALAD

Servings: 8 | Prep: 10m | Cooks: 10m | Total: 20m

NUTRITION FACTS

Calories: 140 | Carbohydrates: 28g | Fat: 2.8g | Protein: 3.5g | Cholesterol: 0mg

INGREDIENTS

- 2 tomatoes, chopped
- 1 large red bell pepper, chopped
- 2 jalapeno peppers, minced
- 3/4 cup lemon juice
- 1 1/4 teaspoons dried cilantro
- 1/4 teaspoon dried basil
- /8 teaspoon red pepper flakes
- 1 (15 ounce) can whole kernel corn; drain and reserve liquid
- 1 (15 ounce) can black beans; drain and reserve liquid
- 1 tablespoon olive oil
- 1/2 cup chopped onion
- 1/2 teaspoon minced garlic
- 1 1/2 cups instant brown rice
- salt and pepper to taste

DIRECTIONS

1. In a large bowl, combine tomatoes, red bell pepper, jalapeno pepper, lemon juice, cilantro, basil, red pepper flakes, corn, and beans. Stir to combine the vegetables, then set aside.
2. In a medium saucepan, heat olive oil at a medium-low heat. Add onions and saute until they are translucent. Add garlic and saute for another minute. Pour in rice and toss to coat. Add reserved liquid from the corn and beans, along with any additional liquid as directed on the rice box. Cook the rice to package specifications. Let the rice cool slightly.
3. Combine the rice and vegetable mixture. Salt and pepper to taste and serve.

SLOW COOKER ROOT VEGETABLE TAGINE

Servings: 8 | Prep: 50m | Cooks: 9h | Total: 9h50m

NUTRITION FACTS

Calories: 131 | Carbohydrates: 31g | Fat: 0.7g | Protein: 2.8g | Cholesterol: 0mg

INGREDIENTS

- 1 pound parsnips, peeled and diced
- 1 pound turnips, peeled and diced
- 2 medium onions, chopped
- 1 pound carrots, peeled and diced
- 6 dried apricots, chopped
- 4 pitted prunes, chopped
- 1 teaspoon ground turmeric
- 1 teaspoon ground cumin
- 1/2 teaspoon ground ginger
- 1/2 teaspoon ground cinnamon
- 1/4 teaspoon ground cayenne pepper
- 1 tablespoon dried parsley
- 1 tablespoon dried cilantro
- 1 (14 ounce) can vegetable broth

DIRECTIONS

1. In a slow cooker, toss together the parsnips, turnips, onions, carrots, apricots, and prunes. Season with turmeric, cumin, ginger, cinnamon, cayenne pepper, parsley, and cilantro. Pour in the vegetable broth.
2. Cover, and cook 9 hours on Low.

RUSH HOUR REFRIED BEANS

Servings: 4 | Prep: 10m | Cooks: 10m | Total: 20m

NUTRITION FACTS

Calories: 68 | Carbohydrates: 12.1g | Fat: 0.6g | Protein: 3.7g | Cholesterol: 0mg

INGREDIENTS

- 2 tablespoons bacon grease
- 2 tablespoons chopped onion
- 1 teaspoon minced garlic
- 1 (15 ounce) can pinto beans, undrained
- 1/4 teaspoon ground cumin

DIRECTIONS

3. Heat bacon grease in a skillet over medium heat. Cook and stir onion and garlic in the hot bacon grease until onions are softened, 5 to 7 minutes. Mash pinto beans and cumin into onion mixture

using a potato masher until reaching your desired consistency. Cook and stir bean mixture until heated through, 3 to 5 minutes.

HOMEMADE SAUERKRAUT

Servings: 8 | Prep: 10m | Cooks: 15m | Total: 25m

NUTRITION FACTS

Calories: 45 | Carbohydrates: 10.2g | Fat: 0.2g | Protein: 2.1g | Cholesterol: 0mg

INGREDIENTS

- 1 cup water
- 1 cup distilled white vinegar, divided
- 1/2 onion, diced
- 1 head cabbage, cored and shredded
- 3/4 teaspoon sea salt
- 1/2 teaspoon celery seed
- 1/2 teaspoon onion powder
- 1/2 teaspoon garlic powder
- ground black pepper to taste

DIRECTIONS

1. Combine water, 1/2 of the vinegar, and onion in a pot over high heat; add cabbage, sea salt, celery seed, onion powder, garlic powder, and black pepper. Pour the remaining vinegar over cabbage mixture. Cover pot and bring water to a boil; cook mixture for about 3 minutes.
2. Stir cabbage mixture and return lid to pot; cook, stirring occasionally, until cabbage is tender and wilted, 10 to 15 minutes more.

CARYN'S CHICKEN

Servings: 4 | Prep: 10m | Cooks: 10m | Total: 20m

NUTRITION FACTS

Calories: 250 | Carbohydrates: 29.9g | Fat: 3.1g | Protein: 27g | Cholesterol: 0mg

INGREDIENTS

- 4 skinless, boneless chicken breast halves - pounded thin
- 6 oranges, juiced
- 3 tablespoons thinly sliced green onion
- ground black pepper to taste

DIRECTIONS

1. Hit the chicken fillets with a tenderizing mallet until they are slightly thinned out.
2. Put the orange juice, green onions and black pepper into a skillet over medium heat. Don't cook over high heat, or the juice will burn and go bitter.
3. Poach the chicken in the juice mixture until it is firm and the juices run clear. This usually takes about 10 minutes, depending on the thickness of the filets. Place the chicken on a serving plate and pour some of the juice mixture on top. Serve.

BREAKFAST BROWNIES

Servings: 12 | Prep: 15m | Cooks: 20m | Total: 40m | Additional: 5m

NUTRITION FACTS

Calories: 129 | Carbohydrates: 20.9g | Fat: 4.1g | Protein: 3.3g | Cholesterol: 16mg

INGREDIENTS

- 1 1/2 cups quick-cooking oats
- 3/4 cup brown sugar
- 3/4 cup flax seed meal
- 1/2 cup gluten-free all purpose baking flour
- 1 teaspoon baking powder
- 1/2 teaspoon ground cinnamon
- 1/4 teaspoon salt
- 1 banana, mashed
- 1/4 cup rice milk
- 1 egg
- 1 teaspoon vanilla extract

DIRECTIONS

1. Preheat oven to 350 degrees F (175 degrees C). Lightly grease an 8x10-inch baking pan.
2. Mix oats, brown sugar, flax seed meal, flour, baking powder, cinnamon, and salt together in a bowl. Mix banana, rice milk, egg, and vanilla extract together in a separate bowl. Pour banana mixture into flour mixture; stir to combine. Pour batter into the prepared baking pan.
3. Bake brownies in the preheated oven until a toothpick inserted in the center comes out clean, about 20 minutes. Cover pan with a towel to hold in moisture and cool brownies for at least 5 minutes before serving.

BBQ CORN

Servings: 10 | Prep: 10m | Cooks: 2h | Total: 10h10m

NUTRITION FACTS

Calories: 121 | Carbohydrates: 20.7g | Fat: 1.1g | Protein: 3.4g | Cholesterol: 0mg

INGREDIENTS

- 10 ears fresh corn with husks
- 1 quart beer
- 1 (7 pound) bag of ice cubes

DIRECTIONS

1. Place whole ears of corn in an ice chest. Pour beer over top. Dump ice out over the ears of corn. Place the lid on the cooler, and let sit 8 hours, or overnight.
2. Preheat smoker to 250 degrees F (120 degrees C).
3. Place corn in the smoker and close the lid. Cook for 1 to 2 hours, turning every 20 minutes or so. Kernels should give easily under pressure when done. To eat, just peel back the husks and use them for a handle.

GINGERY CARROT SALAD

Servings: 6 | Prep: 20m | Cooks: 25m | Total: 45m

NUTRITION FACTS

Calories: 136 | Carbohydrates: 26.4g | Fat: 3.8g | Protein: 1.6g | Cholesterol: 0mg

INGREDIENTS

- 1 pound carrots, cut diagonally into thin slices
- 2 tablespoons cider vinegar
- 1 tablespoon olive oil
- 2 tablespoons Splenda
- 1 clove garlic, grated
- 1/4 teaspoon ground cumin
- 1/4 teaspoon cinnamon
- 1 teaspoon grated fresh ginger
- 1/8 teaspoon seasoned salt
- 1 dash cayenne pepper
- 1/2 cup raisins

DIRECTIONS

1. Bring a large pot of water to boil. Add carrots, and continue to boil until just tender, about 2 minutes. Rinse with cold water, drain well, and set aside.
2. In a large bowl, whisk together the vinegar, olive oil, Splenda, and garlic. Season with cumin, cinnamon, ginger, salt, and cayenne pepper. Stir in carrots and raisins, and toss with dressing. Cover, and refrigerate at least 4 hours.

SLOW COOKER CHICKEN CURRY WITH QUINOA

Servings: 6 | Prep: 30m | Cooks: 4m | Total: 4h30m

NUTRITION FACTS

Calories: 185 | Carbohydrates: 14.4g | Fat: 3.1g | Protein: 24.4g | Cholesterol: 59mg

INGREDIENTS

- 1 1/2 pounds diced chicken breast meat
- 3/4 cup chopped onion
- 1 1/4 cups chopped celery
- 13/4 cups chopped Granny Smith apples
- 1 cup chicken broth
- 1/4 cup nonfat milk
- 1 tablespoon curry powder
- 1/4 teaspoon paprika
- 1/3 cup quinoa

DIRECTIONS

1. Place the chicken, onion, celery, apple, chicken broth, milk, curry powder, and paprika into a slow cooker; stir until mixed. Cover, and cook on Low for 4 to 5 hours. Stir in the quinoa during the final 35 minutes of cooking. Serve when quinoa is tender.

OKRA WITH TOMATOES

Servings: 6 | Prep: 15m | Cooks: 15m | Total: 30m

NUTRITION FACTS

Calories: 66 | Carbohydrates: 13.1g | Fat: 1.1g | Protein: 2.8g | Cholesterol: 0mg

INGREDIENTS

- 1 teaspoon olive oil
- 3 cloves garlic, minced
- 1 pound frozen sliced okra
- 1 (8 ounce) can canned diced tomatoes

- 1 small onion, minced
- 1 teaspoon cayenne pepper
- 1/2 green bell pepper, minced
- 1 (15 ounce) can stewed tomatoes
- salt and ground black pepper to taste

DIRECTIONS

1. Cover the bottom of a skillet with the olive oil and place over medium heat. Place the garlic, onion, and cayenne pepper in the skillet and stir until fragrant. Stir in the green pepper. Cook and stir until tender, about 5 minutes. Stir in the frozen okra and allow to cook for 5 minutes more. Stir in both the diced and the stewed tomatoes. Season with salt and pepper. Reduce heat to medium-low and simmer until all vegetables are tender, 5 to 7 minutes.

SLOW COOKER CARROT CAKE STEEL CUT OATS
Servings: 16 | Prep: 10m | Cooks: 6h | Total: 6h10m

NUTRITION FACTS

Calories: 139 | Carbohydrates: 30.1g | Fat: 1.4g | Protein: 3.1g | Cholesterol: 0mg

INGREDIENTS

- 10 cups water
- 23 ounces unsweetened applesauce
- 2 cups steel cut oats
- 1 (10 ounce) bag shredded carrots
- 1 (8 ounce) can crushed pineapple, drained
- 1 cup raisins
- 1/3 cup granular no-calorie sucralose sweetener (such as Splenda®) (optional)
- 2 tablespoons ground cinnamon
- 1 tablespoon pumpkin pie spice
- 1 teaspoon salt (optional)

DIRECTIONS

1. Combine water, applesauce, oats, carrots, pineapple, raisins, sweetener, cinnamon, pumpkin pie spice, and salt in the crock of a 7-quart or larger slow cooker.
2. Cook on Low for 6 hours.

CB'S BLACK EYED PEAS

Servings: 10 | Prep: 15m | Cooks: 4h10m | Total: 4h25m

NUTRITION FACTS

Calories: 168 | Carbohydrates: 26.1g | Fat: 2.5g | Protein: 11.2g | Cholesterol: 4mg

INGREDIENTS

- 4 slices bacon, chopped
- 1 pound dry black-eyed peas
- 6 cups water
- 1 onion, chopped
- 1 (14.5 ounce) can diced tomatoes, undrained
- 1 jalapeno pepper, finely chopped
- 1 clove garlic, minced
- 1 tablespoon chili powder
- salt to taste
- 1/2 teaspoon lemon pepper

DIRECTIONS

1. Place the bacon in a large, deep skillet, and cook over medium heat, stirring occasionally, until evenly browned, about 10 minutes.
2. Place the dried peas, water, onion, tomatoes, jalapeno pepper, garlic, and chili powder into a slow cooker, and stir to combine. Stir in the bacon and bacon grease, and set the cooker on High. Cook until peas are tender, about 4 hours. Season to taste with salt, and serve.

ROASTED EGGPLANT AND MUSHROOMS

Servings: 2 | Prep: 10m | Cooks: 45m | Total: 55m

NUTRITION FACTS

Calories: 118 | Carbohydrates: 25.8g | Fat: 1.1g | Protein: 6.6g | Cholesterol: 0mg

INGREDIENTS

- 1 medium eggplant, peeled and cubed
- 2 small zucchini, cubed
- 1/2 small yellow onion, chopped
- 1 (8 ounce) package mushrooms, sliced
- 1 1/2 tablespoons tomato paste
- 1/2 cup water
- 1 clove garlic, minced
- 1/2 teaspoon dried basil
- salt and pepper to taste

DIRECTIONS

1. Preheat oven to 450 degrees F (230 degrees C).
2. Place eggplant, zucchini, onion and mushrooms in a 2 quart casserole dish. In a small bowl combine the tomato paste with the water, and stir in garlic, basil, salt and pepper. Pour over the vegetables and mix well.
3. Bake in preheated oven for 45 minutes, or until eggplant is tender, stirring occasionally. Add water as necessary if vegetables begin to stick; however, vegetables should be fairly dry, with slightly browned edges.

CITRUS BROILED ALASKA SALMON

Servings: 8 | Prep: 15m | Cooks: 15m | Total: 30m

NUTRITION FACTS

Calories: 168 | Carbohydrates: 11.6g | Fat: 3.9g | Protein: 21.5g | Cholesterol: 0mg

INGREDIENTS

- 4 large oranges
- 8 (4 ounce) fillets salmon
- 2 teaspoons red wine vinegar
- 1/2 cup chopped green onions
- 2 teaspoons cracked black pepper

DIRECTIONS

1. Preheat the oven's broiler.
2. Slice, peel, and pith oranges; slice crosswise into 1/4 inch rounds. Season fillets with salt. Place salmon fillets on broiling pan.
3. Place the pan of fillets 4 to 6 inches from heat. Cook for 15 minutes under the preheated broiler, or 10 minutes per inch of thickness. Remove from broiler just before they are cooked through. Sprinkle with vinegar. Arrange orange rounds on top. Sprinkle with green onions and cracked black pepper. Broil 1 minute longer.

CHOCOLATE-BANANA TOFU PUDDING

Servings: 4 | Prep: 10m | Cooks: 1h | Total: 1h10m | Additional: 1h

NUTRITION FACTS

Calories: 124 | Carbohydrates: 21.2g | Fat: 3.5g | Protein: 6.1g | Cholesterol: 0mg

INGREDIENTS

- 1 banana, broken into chunks
- 1 (12 ounce) package soft silken tofu
- 1/4 cup confectioners' sugar
- 5 tablespoons unsweetened cocoa powder
- 3 tablespoons soy milk
- 1 pinch ground cinnamon

DIRECTIONS

1. Place the banana, tofu, sugar, cocoa powder, soy milk, and cinnamon into a blender. Cover, and puree until smooth. Pour into individual serving dishes, and refrigerate for 1 hour before serving.

BAR-B-Q BAKED BEANS

Servings: 14 | Prep: 10m | Cooks: 1h | Total: 1h10m

NUTRITION FACTS

Calories: 166 | Carbohydrates: 27g | Fat: 3.3g | Protein: 7.3g | Cholesterol: 5mg

INGREDIENTS

- 1 (15 ounce) can kidney beans, drained (optional)
- 1 (15 ounce) can pinto beans, drained
- 1 (15 ounce) can lima beans, drained
- 1 (16 ounce) can great Northern beans, drained
- 1 (12 ounce) bottle chili sauce
- 2 tablespoons brown sugar
- 1 tablespoon Dijon mustard
- 1 tablespoon Worcestershire sauce
- 2 tablespoons molasses
- 3 slices bacon, cut in half

DIRECTIONS

1. Preheat oven to 325 degrees F (165 degrees C).
2. In a medium baking dish, mix kidney beans, pinto beans, lima beans, great northern beans, chili sauce, brown sugar, Dijon mustard, Worcestershire sauce and molasses. Top with bacon.
3. Bake 1 hour in the preheated oven, until thick and bubbly.

SWEET CARROT SALAD

Servings: 8 | Prep: 10m | Cooks: 30m | Total: 40m

NUTRITION FACTS

Calories: 105 | Carbohydrates: 20.6g | Fat: 2.9g | Protein: 1g | Cholesterol: 1mg

INGREDIENTS

- 1 pound carrots, grated
- 1 cup crushed pineapple
- 1/2 cup raisins
- 1 tablespoon honey
- 2 tablespoons mayonnaise, or to taste
- 1 dash lemon juice

DIRECTIONS

1. In a large bowl, mix together the carrots, pineapple and raisins. Stir in the honey, mayonnaise and lemon juice until evenly coated. Refrigerate for at least 30 minutes before serving to let the flavors meld.

FLORENTINE TOMATO SOUP

Servings: 5 | Prep: 10m | Cooks: 15m | Total: 25m

NUTRITION FACTS

Calories: 54 | Carbohydrates: 8g | Fat: 1.3g | Protein: 3.2g | Cholesterol: < 1mg

INGREDIENTS

- 1 teaspoon olive oil
- 1/2 cup chopped green bell pepper
- 1/2 cup chopped onion
- 1 clove garlic, minced
- 1 (14.5 ounce) can diced tomatoes
- 1 1/2 cups water
- 1 tablespoon minced fresh basil
- 1 teaspoon chicken bouillon granules
- 1/4 teaspoon ground black pepper
- 1 (10 ounce) package frozen chopped spinach, thawed

DIRECTIONS

1. In a large saucepan over medium heat, cook bell pepper, onion and garlic in oil until tender. Stir in tomatoes, water, basil, bouillon and black pepper. Bring to a boil, then reduce heat and simmer 10 minutes.
2. Stir in spinach and cook 5 to 7 minutes more.

ROASTED GRAPES AND CARROTS

Servings: 8 | Prep: 5m | Cooks: 15m | Total: 20m

NUTRITION FACTS

Calories: 140 | Carbohydrates: 26.9g | Fat: 4.2g | Protein: 1.5g | Cholesterol: 0mg

INGREDIENTS

- 2 pounds red seedless grapes
- 1 (16 ounce) package peeled, baby carrots
- 1 medium red onion, cut into wedges
- 2 tablespoons olive oil
- 1 teaspoon ground cumin

DIRECTIONS

1. Preheat oven to 375 degrees F (190 degrees C). Line a baking sheet with aluminum foil.
2. Toss together the grapes, carrots, and red onion in olive oil to coat. Sprinkle with cumin and toss to evenly distribute. Spread mixture on baking sheet.
3. Roast in preheated oven until carrots have begun to soften, about 15 to 20 minutes.

FLORENTINE TOMATO SOUP

Servings: 5 | Prep: 10m | Cooks: 15m | Total: 25m

NUTRITION FACTS

Calories: 54 | Carbohydrates: 8g | Fat: 1.3g | Protein: 3.2g | Cholesterol: < 1mg

INGREDIENTS

- 1 teaspoon olive oil
- 1/2 cup chopped green bell pepper
- 1 1/2 cups water
- 1 tablespoon minced fresh basil

- 1/2 cup chopped onion
- 1 clove garlic, minced
- 1 (14.5 ounce) can diced tomatoes
- 1 teaspoon chicken bouillon granules
- 1/4 teaspoon ground black pepper
- 1 (10 ounce) package frozen chopped spinach, thawed

DIRECTIONS

1. In a large saucepan over medium heat, cook bell pepper, onion and garlic in oil until tender. Stir in tomatoes, water, basil, bouillon and black pepper. Bring to a boil, then reduce heat and simmer 10 minutes.
2. Stir in spinach and cook 5 to 7 minutes more.

VEGETABLE MEDLEY

Servings: 4 | Prep: 20m | Cooks: 15m | Total: 35m

NUTRITION FACTS

Calories: 66 | Carbohydrates: 12.6g | Fat: 1.5g | Protein: 3.3g | Cholesterol: 0mg

INGREDIENTS

- cooking spray
- 1 tomato, diced
- 1 pinch garlic pepper seasoning
- 2 cups fresh mushrooms, sliced
- 2 yellow squash, cubed
- 2 zucchini, cubed

DIRECTIONS

1. Spray a large skillet with cooking spray and add tomatoes. Cook over medium heat for 5 minutes and add garlic pepper. Stir in mushrooms, squash, and zucchini. Simmer until vegetables are tender-crisp, 10 to 15 minutes.

MEXICAN PINTO BEANS

Servings: 12 | Prep: 15m | Cooks: 2h45m | Total: 4h | Additional: 1h

NUTRITION FACTS

Calories: 159 | Carbohydrates: 23g | Fat: 3.2g | Protein: 10.2g | Cholesterol: 10.2mg

INGREDIENTS

- 1 pound dry pinto beans
- 1/2 pound bacon
- 4 serrano peppers

DIRECTIONS

1. Place the beans in a large pot with enough water to cover by 3 to 4 inches, and bring to a boil. Remove from heat, and let sit 1 hour. Drain water. Pour in enough fresh water to cover beans by 3 to 4 inches, and bring to a boil. Reduce heat, cover, and simmer 1 hour.
2. Place bacon in a skillet, and cook over medium high heat until evenly brown. Crumble bacon, and transfer, along with grease, to the pot with the beans. Continue to cook beans on low heat for 30 minutes.
3. Place the whole chile peppers into the pot, and continue cooking beans 1 hour, or until tender.

PUMPKIN SPICE COOKIES

Servings: 56 | Prep: 15m | Cooks: 25m | Total: 28m | Additional: 1m

NUTRITION FACTS

Calories: 74 | Carbohydrates: 12.6g | Fat: 2.2g | Protein: 1.4g | Cholesterol: 8mg

INGREDIENTS

- 2 1/2 cups all-purpose flour
- 2 tablespoons butter
- 1 cup rolled oats
- 1 1/3 cups light brown sugar
- 4 teaspoons baking powder
- 2 eggs
- 1 1/2 teaspoons ground cinnamon
- 1 teaspoon vanilla extract
- 1/2 teaspoon ground nutmeg
- 1 (15 ounce) can pumpkin
- 1 teaspoon pumpkin pie spice
- 1/2 cup apple butter
- 1/2 teaspoon ground ginger
- 1 cup chopped walnuts
- 1/4 teaspoon salt

DIRECTIONS

1. Preheat an oven to 375 degrees F (190 degrees C). Grease 2 baking sheets.

2. Stir the flour, oats, baking powder, cinnamon, nutmeg, pumpkin pie spice, ginger, and salt in a bowl.
3. Beat the butter and brown sugar with an electric mixer in a large bowl until smooth. Add 1 egg and allow it to blend into the mixture before adding the other along with the vanilla. Add the pumpkin and apple butter; continue beating. Mix in the flour mixture until just incorporated. Fold in the walnuts, mixing just enough to evenly combine. Drop spoonfuls of the dough 2 inches apart onto the prepared baking sheets.
4. Bake in the preheated oven until the edges are golden, about 12 minutes. Allow the cookies to cool on the baking sheet for 1 minute before removing to a wire rack to cool completely.

JORGE'S INDIAN-SPICED TOMATO LENTIL SOUP

Servings: 5 | Prep: 15m | Cooks: 20m | Total: 35m

NUTRITION FACTS

Calories: 179 | Carbohydrates: 32.5g | Fat: 1g | Protein: 11.1g | Cholesterol: 2mg

INGREDIENTS

- 4 cups low-sodium vegetable broth, divided
- 1 small yellow onion, finely chopped
- 1 clove garlic, finely chopped
- 1 teaspoon ground coriander
- 1/2 teaspoon ground cinnamon
- 1/8 teaspoon ground turmeric
- 1/8 teaspoon garam masala
- 1/8 teaspoon cayenne pepper
- 1 cup red lentils
- 1 (14.5 ounce) can no-salt-added diced tomatoes, undrained
- 1 tablespoon fresh lemon juice (optional)
- 1 tablespoon crumbled feta cheese (optional)

DIRECTIONS

1. Bring 1/2 cup broth to a boil in a pot; reduce heat and simmer. Add onion and garlic and simmer until onion is translucent and tender, about 5 minutes. Stir coriander, cinnamon, turmeric, garam masala, and cayenne pepper into onion mixture; simmer for 1 minute.
2. Stir lentils into spiced onion mixture; cook, stirring constantly, for 30 seconds. Add remaining 3 1/2 cups broth and tomatoes; bring to a boil. Reduce heat to low, cover, and simmer until lentils are tender, 10 to 12 minutes. Stir lemon juice into soup and garnish with feta cheese.

APPLESAUCE FOR THE FREEZER

Servings: 20 | Prep: 15m | Cooks: 25m | Total: 40m

NUTRITION FACTS

Calories: 63 | Carbohydrates: 16.6g | Fat: 0.1g | Protein: 0.2g | Cholesterol: 0mg

INGREDIENTS

- 3 1/2 pounds apples - peeled, cored, and quartered
- 1 cup water
- 1/4 cup dark brown sugar
- 1/4 cup white sugar, or less to taste
- 3 tablespoons lemon juice, or more to taste
- 1 (3 inch) piece cinnamon stick
- 4 strips lemon zest
- 1/2 teaspoon salt

DIRECTIONS

1. Stir apples, water, brown sugar, white sugar, lemon juice, cinnamon stick, lemon zest, and salt together in a large pot. Place a cover on the pot and bring the mixture to a boil. Reduce heat to medium-low and cook until the apples are soft, 20 to 30 minutes.
2. Remove pot from heat. Remove and discard cinnamon stick and lemon zest strips. Mash apples with a potato masher.

STIR-FRIED SNOW PEAS AND CARROTS

Servings: 2 | Prep: 10m | Cooks: 15m | Total: 25m

NUTRITION FACTS

Calories: 94 | Carbohydrates: 13.4g | Fat: 3g | Protein: 3.9g | Cholesterol: 2mg

INGREDIENTS

- 1 teaspoon soy sauce
- 1 teaspoon cornstarch
- cooking spray
- 1 teaspoon sesame oil
- 1/2 pound snow peas
- 1/2 cup thinly sliced carrot
- 1/2 cup chicken broth
- 1 teaspoon ground cumin

DIRECTIONS

1. Whisk together the soy sauce and cornstarch in a bowl until cornstarch is completely dissolved; set aside.
2. Prepare a skillet with cooking spray and place over medium heat; drizzle in the sesame oil. Place the snow peas and carrots in the skillet; stir-fry for 2 minutes. Pour the broth over the vegetables. Bring to a boil, cover, and reduce heat to low; simmer until vegetables are slightly softened, about 5 minutes. Stir in the soy sauce mixture; continue to stir-fry until the sauce has thickened.

ASPARAGUS GUACAMOLE

Servings: 4 | Prep: 15m | Cooks: 1h | Total: 1h15m

NUTRITION FACTS

Calories: 35 | Carbohydrates: 7.4g | Fat: 0.2g | Protein: 3g | Cholesterol: 0mg

INGREDIENTS

- 24 spears fresh asparagus, trimmed and coarsely chopped
- 1/2 cup salsa
- 1 tablespoon chopped cilantro
- 2 cloves garlic
- 4 green onions, sliced

DIRECTIONS

1. Place the asparagus in a pot with enough water to cover. Bring to a boil, and cook 5 minutes, until tender but firm. Drain, and rinse with cold water.
2. Place the asparagus, salsa, cilantro, garlic, and green onions in a food processor or blender, and process to desired consistency. Refrigerate 1 hour, or until chilled, before serving.

CABBAGE AND RICE

Servings: 8 | Prep: 15m | Cooks: 20m | Total: 35m

NUTRITION FACTS

Calories: 150 | Carbohydrates: 30.4g | Fat: 1.6g | Protein: 4.2g | Cholesterol: 0mg

INGREDIENTS

- 1 cup long grain white rice
- 2 cups water
- 1 clove garlic, crushed
- 1 head cabbage, cored and shredded

- 2 teaspoons olive oil
- 1 medium onion, chopped
- 1 (14.5 ounce) can diced tomatoes
- 1/2 cup jalapeno pepper rings

DIRECTIONS

1. In a saucepan, combine the rice and water. Bring to a boil. Cover and reduce heat to low. Simmer for 15 to 20 minutes, until water is absorbed and rice is tender.
2. Meanwhile, heat the olive oil in a large pot. Add the onion and garlic; cook and stir until fragrant, about 3 minutes. Add the cabbage, and cook for about 10 minutes, stirring occasionally, until the cabbage cooks down. Mix in the tomatoes, pepper rings and cooked rice. Simmer for 10 to 15 minutes to blend the flavors together.

GARBANZO BEAN BURGERS

Servings: 4 | Prep: 30m | Cooks: 30m | Total: 1h30m

NUTRITION FACTS

Calories: 140 | Carbohydrates: 21.7g | Fat: 4.2g | Protein: 4.9g | Cholesterol: 0mg

INGREDIENTS

- 1 (15 ounce) can garbanzo beans, rinsed and drained
- 1 red bell pepper, finely chopped
- 1 carrot, grated
- 3 cloves garlic, minced
- 1 red chile pepper, seeded and minced
- 2 tablespoons chopped fresh cilantro
- 1 tablespoon tahini paste
- salt and black pepper to taste
- 1 teaspoon olive oil (optional)

DIRECTIONS

1. Place garbanzo beans in the bowl of a food processor with bell pepper, carrot, garlic, red chile pepper, cilantro, tahini, salt, and pepper. Place the lid on the food processor, and pulse 5 times, then scrape the sides, and pulse the mixture until it is evenly mixed. If the mixture looks dry, add olive oil.
2. Refrigerate garbanzo bean burger mixture for 30 minutes.
3. Preheat an oven to 350 degrees F (175 degrees C). Prepare a baking sheet with parchment paper or lightly grease with cooking spray.
4. Shape the chilled garbanzo bean burger mixture into patties.
5. Bake 20 minutes, then carefully flip burgers and bake 10 more minutes, or until evenly browned.

GREEN BEANS AND POTATOES

Servings: 6 | Prep: 10m | Cooks: 25m | Total: 35m

NUTRITION FACTS

Calories: 83 | Carbohydrates: 18.3g | Fat: 0.2g | Protein: 2.1g | Cholesterol: 0mg

INGREDIENTS

- 3 cups thinly sliced potatoes
- 2 cups frozen green beans
- 1/2 teaspoon dried thyme
- 1/4 teaspoon ground black pepper
- 1 teaspoon vegetarian Worcestershire sauce
- 1 cup vegetable broth, divided
- 1 teaspoon cornstarch
- 1/4 cup chopped fresh parsley

DIRECTIONS

1. In a large skillet over medium-high heat combine potatoes, green beans, thyme, pepper, Worcestershire sauce and 3/4 cup of broth. Bring to a boil; reduce heat to medium-low, cover and simmer 15 to 20 minutes or until vegetables are tender.
2. In a small bowl blend remaining broth and cornstarch. Stir in parsley; add to potato mixture. Cook, stirring, until bubbly and thickened.

APPLE RAISIN CAKES

Servings: 6 | Prep: 10m | Cooks: 7m | Total: 17m

NUTRITION FACTS

Calories: 203 | Carbohydrates: 41.1g | Fat: 2.1g | Protein: 6.1g | Cholesterol: 62mg

INGREDIENTS

- 2 eggs, beaten
- 1 cup applesauce
- 1 teaspoon ground cinnamon
- 2 teaspoons white sugar
- 1 cup all-purpose flour
- 1/2 cup whole wheat flour
- 2 teaspoons baking powder
- 2 teaspoons vanilla extract
- 1/2 cup raisins

DIRECTIONS

1. In a large mixing bowl, combine eggs, applesauce, cinnamon, sugar, flour, baking powder, vanilla, and raisins. Form small cakes out of the batter.
2. Heat a nonstick griddle over medium heat, fry the cakes until both sides are browned, about 5 to 7 minutes.

FRUIT LEATHER

Servings: 16 | Prep: 20m | Cooks: 5h | Total: 5h20m

NUTRITION FACTS

Calories: 90 | Carbohydrates: 23.5g | Fat: 0.1g | Protein: 0.3g | Cholesterol: 0mg

INGREDIENTS

- 1 cup sugar
- 1/4 cup lemon juice
- 4 cups peeled, cored and chopped apple
- 4 cups peeled, cored and chopped pears

DIRECTIONS

1. Preheat the oven to 150 degrees F (65 degrees C). Cover a baking sheet with a layer of plastic wrap or parchment paper.
2. In the container of a blender, combine the sugar, lemon juice, apple and pear. Cover and puree until smooth. Spread evenly on the prepared pan. Place the pan on the top rack of the oven.
3. Bake for 5 to 6 hours, leaving the door to the oven partway open. Fruit is dry when the surface is no longer tacky and you can tear it like leather. Roll up on the plastic wrap and store in an airtight jar.

SPICY PASTA

Servings: 6 | Prep: 10m | Cooks: 20m | Total: 30m

NUTRITION FACTS

Calories: 134 | Carbohydrates: 22.5g | Fat: 2.8g | Protein: 4.4g | Cholesterol: 0mg

INGREDIENTS

- 1 (12 ounce) package rotini pasta
- 1 tablespoon vegetable oil
- 1 clove garlic, crushed
- 1 onion, diced
- 2 red chile peppers, seeded and chopped
- 1 (14.5 ounce) can diced tomatoes

- 1 teaspoon dried basil
- 1 teaspoon Italian seasoning
- 3 drops hot pepper sauce
- salt and ground black pepper to taste

DIRECTIONS

1. Bring a large pot of lightly salted water to a boil. Cook pasta in boiling water for 8 to 10 minutes, or until al dente; drain.
2. Meanwhile, heat oil in a saucepan over medium heat. Saute garlic with basil and Italian seasoning for 2 to 3 minutes. Stir in onion and chiles; cook until onion is tender. Stir in tomatoes and hot sauce; simmer for 5 minutes, or until heated through. Toss with the cooked pasta, and season with salt and pepper.

THANKSGIVING SPINACH SALAD

Servings: 4 | Prep: 10m | Cooks: 20m | Total: 30m

NUTRITION FACTS

Calories: 115 | Carbohydrates: 30g | Fat: 0.3g | Protein: 1.5g | Cholesterol: 0mg

INGREDIENTS

- 3/4 cup sweetened dried cranberries, chopped
- 1 McIntosh apple - peeled, cored, and diced
- 1/2 small red onion, finely chopped
- 2 tablespoons lemon juice
- 2 teaspoons honey
- 1 teaspoon chili powder
- 1/2 teaspoon ground cinnamon
- 1 (6 ounce) bag baby spinach, torn into bite-sized pieces

DIRECTIONS

1. Mix cranberries, apple, onion, lemon juice, honey, chili powder, and cinnamon together in a large bowl. Let rest for flavors to blend, about 20 minutes. Add spinach and toss to coat.

RUTABAGA OVEN FRIES

Servings: 4 | Prep: 10m | Cooks: 30m | Total: 40m

NUTRITION FACTS

Calories: 50 | Carbohydrates: 8.7g | Fat: 1.4g | Protein: 1.3g | Cholesterol: 0mg

INGREDIENTS

- 1 rutabaga, peeled and cut into spears
- 1 teaspoon olive oil
- 4 sprigs fresh rosemary, minced
- 3 cloves garlic, minced
- 1 pinch salt to taste

DIRECTIONS

1. Preheat oven to 400 degrees F (200 degrees C).
2. Combine rutabaga spears with oil, minced rosemary, garlic, and salt. Toss until evenly coated.
3. Lay rutabaga spears onto a baking sheet, leaving space between for even crisping. Bake until rutabaga fries are cooked through and crisped on the outside, about 30 minutes.

CLASSIC TURKEY AND RICE SOUP

Servings: 6 | Prep: 20m | Cooks: 25m | Total: 45m

NUTRITION FACTS

Calories: 115 | Carbohydrates: 22.4g | Fat: 1.7g | Protein: 3.2g | Cholesterol: 4mg

INGREDIENTS

- 1 turkey carcass
- 1 large onion, halved and skin left on
- 1 large carrot, roughly chopped
- 1 stalk celery, roughly chopped
- 1 head garlic, halved
- 1 teaspoon dried rosemary
- 1 teaspoon dried thyme
- 2 bay leaves
- salt and ground black pepper to taste
- water to cover
- 2 large onions, diced
- 2 carrots, diced
- 2 stalks celery, diced
- 2 cloves garlic, minced
- 1 teaspoon poultry seasoning
- 1 teaspoon dried rosemary
- 1 teaspoon onion powder
- 2 cups cooked rice

DIRECTIONS

1. Combine turkey carcass, halved onion, roughly chopped carrot, roughly chopped celery, halved garlic head, 1 teaspoon rosemary, thyme, bay leaves, salt, and pepper in a stockpot; pour in enough water to cover. Bring mixture to a boil, cover pot, reduce heat, and simmer until flavors have blended, about 1 hour.
2. Remove turkey carcass and pull remaining meat from bones; reserve meat and discard carcass. Remove vegetables and bay leaves from stock using a slotted spoon and discard.
3. Stir diced onions, diced carrots, diced celery, minced garlic, poultry seasoning, 1 teaspoon rosemary, and onion powder into stock; bring to a boil. Reduce heat, cover pot, and simmer until vegetables are very tender, 20 to 30 minutes. Add cooked rice and turkey meat to soup; season with salt and pepper. Cook until rice and turkey meat are warmed, about 5 minutes.

STIR-FRIED MUSHROOMS WITH BABY CORN
Servings: 4 | Prep: 10m | Cooks: 15m | Total: 25m

NUTRITION FACTS

Calories: 49 | Carbohydrates: 8.3g | Fat: 0.9g | Protein: 3.4g | Cholesterol: 0mg

INGREDIENTS

- 2 tablespoons cooking oil
- 3 cloves garlic, minced
- 1 onion, diced
- 8 baby corn ears, sliced
- 2/3 pound fresh mushrooms, sliced
- 1 tablespoon fish sauce
- 1 tablespoon light soy sauce
- 1 tablespoon oyster sauce
- 2 teaspoons cornstarch
- 3 tablespoons water
- 1 red chile pepper, sliced
- 1/4 cup chopped fresh cilantro

DIRECTIONS

1. Heat the oil in a large skillet or wok over medium heat; cook the garlic in the hot oil until browned, 5 to 7 minutes. Add the onion and baby corn and cook until the onion is translucent, 5 to 7 minutes. Add the mushrooms to the mixture and cook until slightly softened, about 2 minutes. Pour the fish sauce, soy sauce, and oyster sauce into the mixture and stir until incorporated.
2. Whisk the cornstarch and water together in a small bowl until the cornstarch is dissolved into the water; pour into the mushroom mixture. Cook and stir until thickened and glistening. Transfer to a serving dish; garnish with the chile pepper and cilantro to serve.

GOURMET MICROWAVE POPCORN

Servings: 2 | Prep: 5m | Cooks: 5m | Total: 10m

NUTRITION FACTS

Calories: 114 | Carbohydrates: 18.5g | Fat: 3.6g | Protein: 3g | Cholesterol: 0mg

INGREDIENTS

- 1/4 cup unpopped popcorn
- salt to taste
- 1 teaspoon olive oil, or more if needed

DIRECTIONS

1. Place popcorn in a brown paper bag. Tightly seal the bag by folding the top several times.
2. Microwave on High until the popping slows, about 2 minutes. Carefully open the bag. Season with salt and drizzle with olive oil. Reclose the bag and shake to distribute the seasoning.

MOROCCAN MASHED POTATOES

Servings: 6 | Prep: 20m | Cooks: 25m | Total: 45m

NUTRITION FACTS

Calories: 103 | Carbohydrates: 21.3g | Fat: 1.4g | Protein: 1.8g | Cholesterol: 0mg

INGREDIENTS

- 10 large baking potatoes, peeled and cubed
- 3 tablespoons olive oil, or as needed
- 1 onion, diced
- 1 tablespoon ground turmeric
- 1 tablespoon salt, or to taste
- 2 teaspoons ground black pepper
- 1/2 teaspoon ground cumin

DIRECTIONS

1. Place the potatoes into a large pot, and fill with enough water to cover. Bring to a boil over medium-high heat, and cook until tender and can be pierced with a fork, about 20 minutes.
2. Meanwhile, place 1 tablespoon olive oil in a skillet, and heat over medium-high heat. Stir in the onion and cook until translucent and lightly browned, about 6 minutes.

3. Drain water from the potatoes, and mash. Stir in the onion, and continue mashing. Mix in the turmeric, salt, pepper, and cumin. Add the remaining 2 tablespoons olive oil, or amount desired to make the potatoes more or less creamy.

BRUSSELS SPROUTS STIR FRY

Servings: 8 | Prep: 20m | Cooks: 15m | Total: 35m

NUTRITION FACTS

Calories: 86 | Carbohydrates: 15.5g | Fat: 2g | Protein: 3.2g | Cholesterol: 0mg

INGREDIENTS

- 1 tablespoon vegetable oil
- 1 onion, chopped
- 1 large potato, peeled and cubed
- 1 bay leaf
- 1 pound Brussels sprouts, trimmed and halved
- 1 red pepper, seeded and cut into 1/2-inch cubes
- 1/4 cup chicken broth
- ground black pepper, to taste
- 2 tablespoons chopped green onions

DIRECTIONS

1. Heat the vegetable oil in a skillet over medium heat. Stir in the onion, potato, and bay leaf. Cook and stir until the onion is transparent, about 5 minutes. Add the Brussels sprouts, red pepper, and chicken broth. Cover and cook until vegetables are tender, about 10 minutes. Remove the bay leaf. Toss with black pepper, to taste. Garnish with green onions, and serve immediately.

HERBED EGGPLANT SLICES

Servings: 4 | Prep: 15m | Cooks: 15m | Total: 30m

NUTRITION FACTS

Calories: 38 | Carbohydrates: 8.7g | Fat: 0.4g | Protein: 1.8g | Cholesterol: 0mg

INGREDIENTS

- 1 clove garlic, minced
- 1 tablespoon minced fresh oregano
- 1 eggplant, sliced into 1/2 inch rounds
- salt to taste

- 1/4 cup chopped fresh basil
- ground black pepper to taste
- 1/2 cup chopped fresh parsley

DIRECTIONS

1. Preheat oven to 400 degrees F (205 degrees C). Coat a baking sheet with cooking spray.
2. In a small bowl, combine garlic, oregano, basil ,and parsley. Mix well, and set aside.
3. Generously season each eggplant slice with salt and pepper on both sides. Place on baking sheet.
4. Bake 5 to 7 minutes on each side, until tender and slightly browned. Sprinkle herb mixture on eggplant slices, and place under the broiler for 30 seconds. Transfer to a serving plate, and serve immediately.

OVEN BAKED TEMPEH

Servings: 6 | Prep: 40m | Cooks: 30m | Total: 1h10m

NUTRITION FACTS

Calories: 118 | Carbohydrates: 13.8g | Fat: 2.8g | Protein: 7.7g | Cholesterol: 0mg

INGREDIENTS

- 1 1/2 teaspoons olive oil
- 2 cups baby carrots, halved
- 1/8 teaspoon crushed red pepper flakes
- 1 cup diced zucchini
- 1 leek, sliced
- 1 (8 ounce) package seasoned tempeh
- 1/3 cup shallots, chopped
- 1/2 cup dry sherry
- 1/2 cup red bell pepper, chopped
- 1 tomato, chopped
- 4 cloves garlic, minced
- 1 tablespoon tamari

DIRECTIONS

1. Preheat oven to 350 degrees F (175 degrees C).
2. Place oil and crushed red pepper in a stovetop-safe and oven proof 2 quart casserole dish. Saute over medium heat for 1 minute. Add leek, shallot, red bell pepper and garlic. Saute for 3 minutes. Add the carrots and zucchini. Saute, stirring frequently for 5 minutes. Add the tempeh and saute for 5 more minutes. Add the sherry, tomato and tamari. Saute for an additional 5 minutes.
3. Cover casserole dish and bake in at 350 degrees F (175 degrees C) for 30 minutes.

CURTIDO (EL SALVADORAN CABBAGE SALAD)

Servings: 4 | Prep: 20m | Cooks: 5m | Total: 45m

NUTRITION FACTS

Calories: 50 | Carbohydrates: 11.3g | Fat: 0.3g | Protein: 2.3g | Cholesterol: 0mg

INGREDIENTS

- 1/2 head green cabbage, cored and shredded
- 1 carrot, grated
- 1 quart boiling water
- 3 green onions, minced
- 1 cup distilled white vinegar
- 1/2 cup water
- teaspoons dried oregano

DIRECTIONS

1. Combine the cabbage and carrot in a large bowl and pour the boiling water over the mixture. Allow the mixture to steep for 5 minutes; drain well. Return the cabbage and carrots to the bowl. Mix in the green onion, vinegar, 1/2 cup of water, and oregano. Toss until all ingredients are combined. Chill for 20 minutes before serving.

SWEET POTATO HUMMUS

Servings: 20 | Prep: 20m | Cooks: 45m | Total: 1h20m

NUTRITION FACTS

Calories: 75 | Carbohydrates: 12.2g | Fat: 2.3g | Protein: 1.6g | Cholesterol: 0mg

INGREDIENTS

- 3 sweet potatoes
- 1 (15 ounce) can garbanzo beans, drained (reserve liquid) and rinsed
- 2 tablespoons extra-virgin olive oil
- 2 tablespoons tahini
- 2 tablespoons lemon juice
- 1/2 teaspoon lemon zest
- 1/4 teaspoon ground cumin
- 1/4 teaspoon ground coriander
- 1/4 teaspoon ground white pepper
- sea salt to taste

DIRECTIONS

1. Preheat oven to 400 degrees F (200 degrees C).
2. Poke holes all over sweet potatoes with a fork.
3. Roast sweet potatoes in the preheated oven until soft, about 45 minutes; let cool. Cut sweet potatoes in half lengthwise.
4. Combine garbanzo beans and olive oil in a blender and pulse several times to mash. Scoop flesh out of sweet potato peels and add to the blender; pulse to combine. Add tahini, lemon juice, lemon zest, cumin, coriander, white pepper, and sea salt to mixture; blend until smooth, adding reserved garbanzo bean liquid as needed to make a smooth, creamy hummus.

FRESH STRAWBERRY GRANITA

Servings: 8 | Prep: 10m | Cooks: 2h15 | Total: 2h25m

NUTRITION FACTS

Calories: 69 | Carbohydrates: 17.1g | Fat: 0.3g | Protein: 0.8g | Cholesterol: 0mg

INGREDIENTS

- 2 pounds ripe strawberries, hulled and halved
- 1/3 cup white sugar, or to taste
- 1 cup water
- 1/2 teaspoon lemon juice (optional)
- 1/4 teaspoon balsamic vinegar (optional)
- 1 tiny pinch salt

DIRECTIONS

1. Rinse strawberries with cold water; let drain. Transfer berries to a blender and add sugar, water, lemon juice, balsamic vinegar, and salt.
2. Pulse several times to get the mixture moving, then blend until smooth, about 1 minute. Pour into a large baking dish. Puree should only be about 3/8 inch deep in the dish.
3. Place dish uncovered in the freezer until mixture barely begins to freeze around the edges, about 45 minutes. Mixture will still be slushy in the center.
4. Lightly stir the crystals from the edge of the granita mixture into the center, using a fork, and mix thoroughly. Close freezer and chill until granita is nearly frozen, 30 to 40 more minutes. Mix lightly with a fork as before, scraping the crystals loose. Repeat freezing and stirring with the fork 3 to 4 times until the granita is light, crystals are separate, and granita looks dry and fluffy.
5. Portion granita into small serving bowls to serve.

OVEN BAKED TEMPEH

Servings: 6 | Prep: 20m | Cooks: 25m | Total: 45m

NUTRITION FACTS

Calories: 118 | Carbohydrates: 13.8g | Fat: 2.8g | Protein: 7.7g | Cholesterol: 0mg

INGREDIENTS

- 1 1/2 teaspoons olive oil
- 1/8 teaspoon crushed red pepper flakes
- 1 leek, sliced
- 1/3 cup shallots, chopped
- 1/2 cup red bell pepper, chopped
- 4 cloves garlic, minced
- 2 cups baby carrots, halved
- 1 cup diced zucchini
- 1 (8 ounce) package seasoned tempeh
- 1/2 cup dry sherry
- 1 tomato, chopped
- 1 tablespoon tamari

DIRECTIONS

1. Preheat oven to 350 degrees F (175 degrees C).
2. Place oil and crushed red pepper in a stovetop-safe and oven proof 2 quart casserole dish. Saute over medium heat for 1 minute. Add leek, shallot, red bell pepper and garlic. Saute for 3 minutes. Add the carrots and zucchini. Saute, stirring frequently for 5 minutes. Add the tempeh and saute for 5 more minutes. Add the sherry, tomato and tamari. Saute for an additional 5 minutes.
3. Cover casserole dish and bake in at 350 degrees F (175 degrees C) for 30 minutes.

EASY ROASTED POTATOES

Servings: 6 | Prep: 15m | Cooks: 40m | Total: 55m

NUTRITION FACTS

Calories: 128 | Carbohydrates: 24.6 g | Fat: 2.5g | Protein: 3g | Cholesterol: 0mg

INGREDIENTS

- 1 teaspoon McCormick® Dill Weed
- 1 teaspoon McCormick® Garlic Powder
- 1/2 teaspoon salt
- 1/4 teaspoon McCormick® Black Pepper, Coarse Ground
- 2 pounds red potatoes, cut into wedges
- 1 tablespoon olive oil

DIRECTIONS

1. Preheat oven to 400 degrees F. Mix dill weed, garlic powder, salt and pepper in small bowl. Set aside.
2. Toss potatoes with oil in large bowl. Sprinkle seasoning mixture over potatoes; toss to coat.
3. Spread potatoes in single layer on foil-lined 15x10x1-inch baking pan.
4. Bake 40 minutes or until potatoes are tender and golden brown.

POTATO SALAD

Servings: 4 | Prep: 40m | Cooks: 10m | Total: 50m

NUTRITION FACTS

Calories: 104 | Carbohydrates: 23.6g | Fat: 0.3g | Protein: 2.6g | Cholesterol: <1mg

INGREDIENTS

- 2 potatoes
- 2 tablespoons low-fat mayonnaise
- 2 tablespoons fat free ranch dressing
- 1/4 onion, chopped
- 1 stalk celery
- 1 green bell pepper, chopped
- salt and pepper to taste

DIRECTIONS

1. Bring a pot of salted water to boil, place potatoes in water. Boil until potatoes are tender. Drain well. Let the potatoes cool 30 minutes.
2. Peel the skin off of the potatoes and cube them.
3. In a medium size mixing bowl combine potatoes, mayonnaise, ranch dressing, onion, celery, green pepper, salt and pepper. Cover and refrigerate until well chilled.

SEAFOOD GUMBO STOCK

Servings: 8 | Prep: 15m | Cooks: 7h35m | Total: 7h50m

NUTRITION FACTS

Calories: 112 | Carbohydrates: 12.1g | Fat: 1.3g | Protein: 13.2g | Cholesterol: 86mg

INGREDIENTS

- shells from 1 pound shrimp
- 5 quarts water
- 4 carrots, sliced
- 4 onions, quartered
- 1/2 bunch celery, sliced
- 2 bay leaves
- 3 cloves garlic, sliced
- 2 sprigs fresh parsley
- 5 whole cloves
- 1 teaspoon ground black pepper
- 1 tablespoon dried basil
- 2 teaspoons dried thyme

DIRECTIONS

1. Bake shrimp shells at 375 degrees F (195 degrees C) until dried and starting to brown on edges.
2. In an 8-quart pot, combine water, carrots, onions, celery, bay leaves, garlic, parsley, cloves, pepper, basil, thyme and shrimp shells. Bring slowly to a boil.
3. Reduce heat, and cook 5 to 7 hours. Replace water as needed, 2 or 3 times, by pouring more water down the inside of the pot.
4. Remove stock from heat, and strain. Press all liquid from the shells and vegetables, then discard them. Return liquid to heat, and reduce to 2 to 3 quarts, or to taste.

FISH SINIGANG (TILAPIA) - FILIPINO SOUR BROTH DISH

Servings: 4 | Prep: 5m | Cooks: 10m | Total: 15m

NUTRITION FACTS

Calories: 112 | Carbohydrates: 13.4g | Fat: 1g | Protein: 13.1g | Cholesterol: 21mg

INGREDIENTS

- 1/2 pound tilapia fillets, cut into chunks
- 1 small head bok choy, chopped
- 2 medium tomatoes, cut into chunks
- 1 cup thinly sliced daikon radish
- 1/4 cup tamarind paste
- 3 cups water
- 2 dried red chile peppers (optional)

DIRECTIONS

1. In a medium pot, combine the tilapia, bok choy, tomatoes and radish. Stir together the tamarind paste and water; pour into the pot. Toss in the chili peppers if using. Bring to a boil, and cook for 5 minutes, or just until the fish is cooked through. Even frozen fish will cook in less than 10 minutes. Do not over cook or else the fish will fall apart. Ladle into bowls to serve.

MICROWAVE CORN-ON-THE-COB IN THE HUSK

Servings: 1 | Prep: 5m | Cooks: 5m | Total: 10m

NUTRITION FACTS

Calories: 77 | Carbohydrates: 17.1g | Fat: 1.1g | Protein: 2.9g | Cholesterol: 0mg

INGREDIENTS

- 1 ear fresh corn in the husk

DIRECTIONS

1. Rinse entire ear of corn under water briefly. Wrap corn in a paper towel and place on a microwave-safe plate.
2. Cook corn in the microwave oven until hot and cooked through, 3 to 5 minutes. Remove from microwave and let rest for 2 minutes. Remove corn husk.

OVEN FRIED OKRA

Servings: 4 | Prep: 10m | Cooks: 25m | Total: 35m

NUTRITION FACTS

Calories: 95 | Carbohydrates: 19.1g | Fat: 2g | Protein: 3.3g | Cholesterol: 0mg

INGREDIENTS

- 1 (16 ounce) package frozen cut okra
- butter flavored cooking spray
- 1/4 cup yellow cornmeal
- 1/4 cup panko bread crumbs
- 1/2 teaspoon garlic salt
- 1/4 teaspoon ground black pepper (optional)

DIRECTIONS

1. Preheat an oven to 375 degrees F (190 degrees C). Place a baking rack on top of a baking sheet or sheet pan.
2. Cook the frozen okra in the microwave using your microwave's frozen vegetable setting, or on high for 8 minutes. Drain and cool on paper towels, about 5 to 10 minutes. Spray generously with butter flavored cooking spray. Add the cornmeal, panko bread crumbs, garlic salt, and pepper to a plastic food storage bag. Place the okra into the bag and shake to coat the okra with the cornmeal mixture.
3. Remove the okra from the bag and spread it on the prepared baking rack. Bake in the preheated oven until golden brown and crispy, about 15 to 20 minutes.

GRILLED ASIAN ASPARAGUS

Servings: 5 | Prep: 5m | Cooks: 5m | Total: 40m

NUTRITION FACTS

Calories: 84 | Carbohydrates: 15.1g | Fat: 1.9g | Protein: 3.2g | Cholesterol: 0mg

INGREDIENTS

- 1 pound fresh asparagus, trimmed
- 1/2 cup hoisin sauce
- sesame seeds

DIRECTIONS

1. Place asparagus and hoisin sauce into a resealable plastic bag and shake several times to coat asparagus with sauce. Allow to stand at least 30 minutes. For best flavor, refrigerate and marinate overnight.
2. Preheat an outdoor grill for medium heat and lightly oil the grate.
3. Remove asparagus from bag and shake off excess hoisin sauce; lay asparagus spears onto the grill and cook, turning every 1 to 2 minutes, until all sides of the spears show grill marks and hoisin sauce has caramelized onto the asparagus, 4 to 6 minutes.
4. Transfer asparagus to a serving platter and sprinkle with sesame seeds to serve.

SAUTEED KALE WITH APPLES

Servings: 4 | Prep: 15m | Cooks: 15m | Total: 30m

NUTRITION FACTS

Calories: 123 | Carbohydrates: 21.6g | Fat: 4g | Protein: 3g | Cholesterol: 0mg

INGREDIENTS

- 1 tablespoon olive oil
- 1 white onion, sliced
- 2 Red Delicious apples, cored and cut into bite-size pieces
- 2 teaspoons apple cider vinegar
- 1/8 teaspoon sea salt
- 1/8 teaspoon ground black pepper
- 4 cups chopped kale leaves

DIRECTIONS

1. Heat olive oil in a large skillet over medium heat; cook and stir onion until tender, about 4 minutes. Add apples, vinegar, salt, and pepper; cover skillet and cook until apples are tender, about 3 minutes. Add kale; cover and cook until kale is tender, 4 to 5 minutes.

ZUCCHINI-TOMATO SAUTE

Servings: 15 | Prep: 20m | Cooks: 1h | Total: 1h20m

NUTRITION FACTS

Calories: 92 | Carbohydrates: 9.9g | Fat: 1g | Protein: 13.2g | Cholesterol: 22mg

INGREDIENTS

- 8 tilapia fillets
- 15 limes, juiced
- 1 large tomato, finely diced
- salt and pepper to taste
- 1 large red onion, finely diced
- 2 cucumbers, peeled, seeded, and finely diced
- 1/2 bunch finely chopped cilantro

DIRECTIONS

1. Chop the raw tilapia into small pieces, and place in a large bowl. Pour in enough lime juice to cover the fish.
2. Mix the tomato, red onion, and cucumbers into the bowl. Stir in the cilantro. Season with salt and pepper.
3. Allow the ceviche to marinate, refrigerated, for at least an hour. Taste for seasoning before serving; add salt and pepper if necessary.

CHICKEN GUMBO SOUP

Servings: 8 | Prep: 10m | Cooks: 3h20m | Total: 3h30m

NUTRITION FACTS

Calories: 116 | Carbohydrates: 20.5g | Fat: 0.7g | Protein: 7.5g | Cholesterol: 9mg

INGREDIENTS

- 8 cups water
- 1 teaspoon garlic powder
- 1 tablespoon hot pepper sauce
- 2 carrots, sliced thin
- 4 ounces fresh mushrooms
- 1 (10 ounce) package frozen okra, thawed and sliced
- 1/4 cup uncooked wild rice
- 1 skinless, boneless chicken breast half - cut into cubes
- 1 1/2 cups uncooked rotini pasta
- salt to taste
- ground black pepper to taste
- 3 green onions, thinly sliced

DIRECTIONS

1. Bring the water to a boil. Add the garlic powder and the hot pepper sauce. Put the carrots and mushrooms into the pot of water. Cook for five minutes.
2. Add the okra, wild rice, and chicken cubes. Turn heat to low, and cook for three hours.
3. Add the spiral pasta, and cook for ten minutes. Add salt and pepper to taste. Serve hot, garnished with green onions.

CHLOE'S QUICK FRUIT SALAD

Servings: 4 | Prep: 15m | Cooks: 30m | Total: 45m

NUTRITION FACTS

Calories: 90 | Carbohydrates: 20.6g | Fat: 0.7g | Protein: 2.3g | Cholesterol: 1mg

INGREDIENTS

- 1 apple, cored and chopped
- 1 large orange, peeled, sectioned, and cut into bite-size
- 1/2 cup seedless grapes
- 1 nectarine, pitted and chopped
- 1/4 cup fresh orange juice
- 6 tablespoons plain low-fat yogurt

DIRECTIONS

1. In a mixing bowl, combine the apple, orange, grapes and nectarine. If using a passion fruit, spoon out the flesh and chop.
2. Pour enough fresh juice to coat and prevent oxidation. Toss and refrigerate.
3. Serve with dollop of low-fat yogurt.

MANHATTAN CLAM CHOWDER
Servings: 8 | Prep: 20m | Cooks: 25m | Total: 45m

NUTRITION FACTS

Calories: 82 | Carbohydrates: 15.8g | Fat: 0.2g | Protein: 3.9g | Cholesterol: 5mg

INGREDIENTS

- 1 pint shucked clams
- 1 cup tomato and clam juice cocktail
- 2 potatoes, cleaned and chopped
- 1 cup chopped green bell pepper
- 1/4 cup chopped green onions
- 1/4 teaspoon ground black pepper
- 1 (14.5 ounce) can Italian-style diced tomatoes

DIRECTIONS

1. Chop clams, reserving juice; set clams aside. Strain clam juice to remove bits of shell. Measure juice; add enough water to equal 1 1/2 cups liquid.
2. Combine clam juice mixture, clam-tomato juice cocktail, potatoes, bell peppers, scallions and black pepper in large saucepan; heat to a boil. Reduce heat; cover and simmer for about 15 minutes or until potatoes are just tender.
3. Stir in the undrained tomatoes and the chopped clams and heat through.

BANGAN KA BHURTA (INDIAN EGGPLANT)
Servings: 4 | Prep: 15m | Cooks: 15m | Total: 35m

NUTRITION FACTS

Calories: 61 | Carbohydrates: 11.8g | Fat: 1.5g | Protein: 2g | Cholesterol: 0mg

INGREDIENTS

- 1 eggplant
- 1 teaspoon vegetable oil
- 1 medium onion, chopped
- 2 roma (plum) tomatoes, chopped
- 1/4 teaspoon ground cayenne pepper
- 1/4 teaspoon salt
- 1/4 teaspoon pepper
- 4 sprigs chopped fresh cilantro

DIRECTIONS

1. Preheat the oven broiler. Place eggplant in a roasting pan, and broil 5 minutes, turning occasionally, until about 1/2 the skin is scorched.
2. Place eggplant in microwave safe dish. Cook 5 minutes on High in the microwave, or until tender. Cool enough to handle, and remove skin, leaving some scorched bits. Cut into thick slices.
3. Heat oil in a skillet over medium heat, stir in the onion, and cook until tender. Mix in eggplant, and tomatoes. Season with cayenne pepper, salt, and black pepper. Continue to cook and stir until soft. Garnish with cilantro to serve.

MEXICAN HOT CARROTS

Servings: 8 | Prep: 15m | Cooks: 15m | Total: 8h30m

NUTRITION FACTS

Calories: 45 | Carbohydrates: 10.5g | Fat: 0.2g | Protein: 1.1g | Cholesterol: 0mg

INGREDIENTS

- 6 carrots, peeled and sliced
- 2 onions, thinly sliced
- 1 (16 ounce) jar sliced jalapeno peppers, with liquid
- 1 cup vinegar

DIRECTIONS

1. Place the carrots in a saucepan with enough water to cover and cook over medium heat until nearly boiling, 7 to 10 minutes. Immediately drain the carrots and set aside to cool.
2. Divide the cooled carrots into two 1-quart glass jars. Alternate layers of onion and jalapeno peppers atop the carrots until the jars are full.
3. Mix the liquid from the jalapeno peppers and the vinegar in a saucepan; bring the mixture to a rolling boil. Remove from heat and pour the liquid into the jars until full. Seal the jars with lids. Place the jars in the refrigerator until cold, at least 8 hours.

ITALIAN ROASTED CAULIFLOWER

Servings: 4 | Prep: 25m | Cooks: 30m | Total: 1h55m

NUTRITION FACTS

Calories: 90 | Carbohydrates: 14.7g | Fat: 2.7g | Protein: 3.7g | Cholesterol: 0mg

INGREDIENTS

- 1 head cauliflower, cut into florets
- 1 large red bell pepper, cut into 1-1/2 inch pieces
- 1 red onion, sliced
- 1/2 cup chopped fresh dill
- 3 tablespoons balsamic vinegar
- 2 tablespoons white wine vinegar
- 2 teaspoons olive oil
- salt and pepper to taste

DIRECTIONS

1. Combine the cauliflower, bell pepper, onion, dill, balsamic vinegar, white wine vinegar, and olive oil in a large resalable bag; shake bag to evenly coat. Allow to marinate in refrigerator 1 to 2 hours, turning bag occasionally.
2. Preheat oven to 450 degrees F (230 degrees C).
3. Open the bag and season with salt and pepper; reseal the bag and shake again to coat. Pour into a 9x13 glass baking dish.
4. Bake in the preheated oven until tender, about 30 minutes, stirring occasionally.

SQUASH AND GREEN BEAN SAUTE SIDE DISH

Servings: 2 | Prep: 15m | Cooks: 10m | Total: 25m

NUTRITION FACTS

Calories: 89 | Carbohydrates: 19.6g | Fat: 0.9g | Protein: 5.1g | Cholesterol: 0mg

INGREDIENTS

- 2 yellow squash, sliced
- 1 1/2 cups green beans
- 1 1/2 cups halved cherry tomatoes
- 2 tablespoons fresh lemon juice
- 1 tablespoon dried parsley
- 1/2 teaspoon ground coriander
- 1/8 teaspoon salt, or to taste
- 1/8 teaspoon ground black pepper, or to taste

DIRECTIONS

1. Cook and stir squash and green beans in a nonstick skillet over medium heat until slightly softened, 2 to 3 minutes. Stir tomatoes, lemon juice, parsley, coriander, salt, and black pepper into squash mixture; cook and stir until tomatoes have softened, 5 to 10 minutes.

CURRIED COTTAGE FRIES

Servings: 8 | Prep: 10m | Cooks: 20m | Total: 30m

NUTRITION FACTS

Calories: 162 | Carbohydrates: 28.5g | Fat: 4.1g | Protein: 3.8g | Cholesterol: <1mg

INGREDIENTS

- 6 potatoes, cut into wedges
- 2 tablespoons vegetable oil
- 2 tablespoons shredded Parmesan cheese
- 2 teaspoons curry powder
- 1 teaspoon paprika
- 1 teaspoon salt
- 1/2 teaspoon garlic powder

DIRECTIONS

4. Preheat oven to 400 degrees F (200 degrees C). Grease a baking sheet.

1. Place potatoes, vegetable oil, Parmesan cheese, curry powder, paprika, salt, and garlic powder in a resealable plastic bag; shake to coat. Spread seasoned potatoes over prepared baking sheet.
2. Bake in preheated oven until tender, about 20 minutes.

TOMATO AND ZUCCHINI MELANGE

Servings: 2 | Prep: 5m | Cooks: 5m | Total: 10m

NUTRITION FACTS

Calories: 47 | Carbohydrates: 10.2g | Fat: 0.6g | Protein: 3g | Cholesterol: 0mg

INGREDIENTS

- 2 plum tomatoes, halved and cut into 1/4 inch slices
- 1 large zucchini, sliced
- 1/2 teaspoon dried oregano
- 1/4 teaspoon dried basil

- 3 tablespoons salsa

- 3 tablespoons water

- salt and pepper to taste

DIRECTIONS

1. In a small saucepan, mix together tomatoes, zucchini, salsa, water, oregano, basil, salt, and pepper. Mix in bell peppers if desired. Bring to a boil over medium heat, then reduce to a simmer. Simmer 3 to 4 minutes, stirring frequently.

MILLET-STUFFED PEPPERS
Servings: 5 | Prep: 10m | Cooks: 25m | Total: 35m

NUTRITION FACTS

Calories: 189 | Carbohydrates: 37.6g | Fat: 2.1g | Protein: 6.1g | Cholesterol: 0mg

INGREDIENTS

- 1 cup millet

- 4 cups water

- 4 cubes vegetable bouillon

- 5 medium bell peppers

- 3 medium tomatoes, chopped

- 1 (15 ounce) can black beans, drained

DIRECTIONS

1. Combine the millet, water and vegetable bouillon in a saucepan, and bring to a boil. Reduce heat to low, cover, and simmer for 15 minutes, or until the water is absorbed.
2. Slice the tops off of the peppers, and remove the seeds and cores. Set aside. When the millet is done, stir in the tomatoes and black beans. Spoon into the peppers until filled. Place the peppers into a glass baking dish, and cover with plastic wrap.
3. Cook in the microwave for 10 minutes, or until peppers are tender. Turn peppers every 2 to 3 minutes to ensure even cooking.

SLOW COOKER CHOCOLATE BANANA STEEL CUT OATS
Servings: 12 | Prep: 5m | Cooks: 6h | Total: 6h5m

NUTRITION FACTS

Calories: 180 | Carbohydrates: 36.9g | Fat: 2.6g | Protein: 6g | Cholesterol: 0mg

INGREDIENTS

- cooking spray
- 10 cups water
- 2 cups steel-cut oats
- 2 pounds ripe bananas, mashed
- 1/2 cup unsweetened cocoa powder
- 1/3 cup granular no-calorie sucralose sweetener (such as Splenda®) (optional)

DIRECTIONS

1. Lightly spray a 5-quart or larger slow cooker crock with cooking spray.
2. Mix water, oats, mashed bananas, cocoa powder, and sweetener in prepared slow cooker.
3. Cook on Low for 6 hours.

FRIED YELLOW SQUASH

Servings: 4 | Prep: 10m | Cooks: 15m | Total: 25m

NUTRITION FACTS

Calories: 130 | Carbohydrates: 21.2g | Fat: 4g | Protein: 3g | Cholesterol: <1mg

INGREDIENTS

- 3/4 cup self-rising cornbread mix (such as Martha White®)
- salt and ground black pepper to taste
- 2 yellow squash, cut into 1/8-inch slices
- 1/4 cup olive oil, or more as needed

DIRECTIONS

1. Place cornbread mix in a gallon-size resealable bag; season with salt and black pepper. Add squash, seal bag, and shake to coat evenly. Remove squash from bag and shake off any excess cornmeal.
2. Heat about 1/4 inch of olive oil in a large skillet over medium heat. Fry squash in the hot oil, working in batches, until center is cooked and edges are crisp, 2 to 3 minutes per side. Remove with a slotted spoon and drain on a paper towel-lined plate.

PAT'S BAKED OATMEAL

Servings: 15 | Prep: 15m | Cooks: 25m | Total: 40m

Calories: 224 | Carbohydrates: 39.7g | Fat: 4.3g | Protein: 7.7g | Cholesterol: 44mg

INGREDIENTS

- 6 cups rolled oats
- 4 eggs, beaten
- 2 cups frozen blueberries
- 1 cup applesauce
- 1 cup brown sugar
- 2 cups skim milk
- 1/4 cup flax seed meal (optional)
- 3 tablespoons wheat germ (optional)
- 1 tablespoon baking powder
- 1 tablespoon ground cinnamon
- 2 teaspoons vanilla extract
- 1/2 teaspoon salt

DIRECTIONS

1. Preheat oven to 350 degrees F (175 degrees C).
2. Mix oats, eggs, blueberries, applesauce, brown sugar, skim milk, flax seed meal, wheat germ, baking powder, cinnamon, vanilla, and salt together in a large bowl; pour into a 9x13-inch baking dish.
3. Bake in preheated oven until the moisture is absorbed and the oats are tender, 25 to 32 minutes.

SUGAR-FREE AND DAIRY-FREE SLOW COOKER STEEL-CUT OATMEAL

Servings: 6 | Prep: 10m | Cooks: 3h | Total: 3h10m

NUTRITION FACTS

Calories: 159 | Carbohydrates: 32.8g | Fat: 1.8g | Protein: 4g | Cholesterol: 0mg

INGREDIENTS

- 2 bananas, mashed
- 5 cups water, divided
- 1 cup steel cut oats
- 1/4 cup raisins (optional)
- 1 teaspoon cinnamon
- 1 teaspoon vanilla extract

DIRECTIONS

1. Put bananas into a blender with 1 cup water; puree and pour into a slow cooker. Add remaining water, oats, raisins, cinnamon, and vanilla extract.
2. Cook on Medium, stirring every 30 minutes, for 3 hours.

YELLOW SQUASH AND ZUCCHINI DELIGHT

Servings: 4 | Prep: 15m | Cooks: 25m | Total: 40m

NUTRITION FACTS

Calories: 63 | Carbohydrates: 12.3g | Fat: 0.3g | Protein: 4.8g | Cholesterol: 0mg

INGREDIENTS

- 1 zucchini, sliced
- 1 yellow squash, sliced
- 1/2 small head cabbage, sliced
- 1 large onion, sliced
- 1 (14.5 ounce) can fat-free chicken broth

DIRECTIONS

1. In a large pot place zucchini, yellow squash, cabbage and onion. Pour broth over vegetables and bring to a boil over medium heat. Reduce heat to low, cover and simmer for 20 to 30 minutes.

TABBOULEH

Servings: 11 | Prep: 20m | Cooks: 1h30m | Total: 1h50m

NUTRITION FACTS

Calories: 118 | Carbohydrates: 18.9g | Fat: 4.2g | Protein: 3.3g | Cholesterol: 0mg

INGREDIENTS

- 1 1/2 cups bulgur
- 3 cups boiling water
- 2 pounds tomatoes, diced
- 1 cup chopped fresh parsley
- 3 green onions, minced
- 1/4 cup minced fresh mint leaves
- 3 tablespoons olive oil
- 1/4 cup fresh lemon juice
- salt to taste
- ground black pepper to taste

DIRECTIONS

1. Place bulgur in a casserole dish, and cover it with 3 cups boiling water. Cover. Let stand 30 minutes, or until the water has been absorbed.
2. Fluff bulgur with a fork. Add tomatoes, parsley, green onions, mint, olive oil, lemon juice, salt and pepper; stir to combine. Cover, and refrigerate for 1 to 2 hours. Serve either chilled or at room temperature.

BANANA OAT AND BRAN COOKIES
Servings: 5 | Prep: 5m | Cooks: 10m | Total: 15m

NUTRITION FACTS

Calories: 117 | Carbohydrates: 27.6g | Fat: 0.5g | Protein: 2.7g | Cholesterol: 1mg

INGREDIENTS

- 2 ripe bananas, mashed
- 1/2 cup whole wheat flour
- 1/4 cup wheat bran
- 1/4 cup rolled oats
- 1/2 cup packed brown sugar
- 1/2 cup low-fat plain yogurt
- 1/5 cup real maple syrup
- 2 egg whites
- 1 teaspoon ground cinnamon
- 1/2 teaspoon salt
- 1/2 teaspoon baking powder
- 1/2 cup raisins

DIRECTIONS

1. Preheat oven to 350 degrees F (175 degrees C).
2. Beat mashed bannanas, egg whites, brown sugar, maple syrup, yogurt, and cinnamon.
3. Combine the remaining dry ingredients: flour, oats, wheat bran, salt and baking powder in a separate bowl. Use an electric mixer to combine dry ingredients with wet mixture.
4. Add in raisins, chopped prunes, and/ or nuts.
5. Roll cookies into balls, place on a cookie sheet coated with cooking spray. Bake for 8-12 minutes until cookies are firm and dry.

WARM CHICKEN AND MANGO SALAD

Servings: 4 | Prep: 15m | Cooks: 15m | Total: 30m

NUTRITION FACTS

Calories: 275 | Carbohydrates: 29.9g | Fat: 4.3g | Protein: 30.8g | Cholesterol: 69mg

INGREDIENTS

- 1/3 cup vanilla low-fat yogurt
- 1 1/2 tablespoons lime juice
- 1 1/2 tablespoons mango chutney
- 1 tablespoon seasoned rice vinegar
- 1 teaspoon honey
- 1/4 teaspoon ground cumin
- 1/4 teaspoon ground coriander
- 1/4 teaspoon ground paprika
- 1 teaspoon olive oil
- 4 skinless, boneless chicken breast halves - cut into strips
- 2 teaspoons grated fresh ginger
- 1 clove garlic, peeled and minced
- 1 1/2 cups peeled, seeded and chopped mango
- 1 cup sliced red bell pepper
- 1/3 cup chopped green onion
- 8 cups torn romaine lettuce

DIRECTIONS

1. In a small bowl, blend vanilla yogurt, lime juice, mango chutney, rice vinegar, honey, cumin, coriander, and paprika.
2. Heat olive oil in a medium skillet over medium heat. Place chicken, ginger, and garlic in the skillet. Cook 7 to 10 minutes, stirring occasionally, until chicken is no longer pink and juices run clear.
3. Mix mango, red bell pepper, and green onions into the skillet. Cook about 5 minutes, until pepper is tender and mangoes are heated through. Stir in the vanilla yogurt mixture. Spoon over romaine lettuce to serve.

FRIJOLES

Servings: 12 | Prep: 10m | Cooks: 5h | Total: 5h10m

NUTRITION FACTS

Calories: 156 | Carbohydrates: 24.9g | Fat: 2.6 g | Protein: 8.3g | Cholesterol: 2mg

INGREDIENTS

- 1 pound dried pinto beans, washed
- 1 white onion, chopped
- 1/2 bunch fresh cilantro, chopped
- 1 fresh jalapeno pepper, chopped
- 3 cloves garlic, minced
- 2 tablespoons lard
- water to cover
- salt to taste

DIRECTIONS

1. Place beans in a large pot with onion, cilantro, jalapeno pepper, garlic, and lard; add enough water to cover with 4 to 5 inches of water. Bring to a boil, reduce heat, and cook for 2 to 3 hours. Depending on the beans, it may take up to 5 hours. Add more water if necessary.
2. When beans are soft, season to taste with salt.

SECRET INGREDIENT PICO DE GALLO

Servings: 4 | Prep: 20m | Cooks: 1h | Total: 1h20m

NUTRITION FACTS

Calories: 49 | Carbohydrates: 10.9g | Fat: 0.5g | Protein: 2.2g | Cholesterol: 0mg

INGREDIENTS

- 1/2 cup minced onion
- 2 jalapeno peppers, seeded and minced
- 1/4 cup diced red bell pepper
- 1/4 cup minced dill pickle
- 4 large tomatoes, seeded and diced
- 1 tablespoon fresh lime juice
- 1/4 cup chopped cilantro
- salt and pepper to taste

DIRECTIONS

1. In a medium bowl, combine the onion, jalapeno pepper, bell pepper, dill pickle, and diced tomatoes. Stir in lime juice and cilantro; season to taste with salt and pepper. Cover, and refrigerate at least 1 hour before serving, preferably overnight.

CHICKEN SOUP WITH ADZUKI BEANS, ESCAROLE, AND SWEET POTATO

Servings: 12 | Prep: 15m | Cooks: 2h | Total: 2h15m

NUTRITION FACTS

Calories: 169 | Carbohydrates: 29.1g | Fat: 1.9g | Protein: 9.9g | Cholesterol: 14mg

INGREDIENTS

- 1 1/2 quarts chicken broth
- 4 boneless, skinless chicken thighs
- 1 cup dry adzuki beans
- 1 cup uncooked wild rice
- 2 onions, cut into large chunks
- 1 tablespoon bottled minced garlic
- 1 teaspoon dried sage
- 1 tablespoon dried thyme
- 1 tablespoon dried rosemary
- 1 large sweet potato, peeled and cubed
- 1 zucchini, cubed
- 1 yellow squash, cubed
- 1/3 medium head escarole, coarsely chopped

DIRECTIONS

1. Place the chicken broth in a large pot. Mix in the chicken thighs, adzuki beans, wild rice, onions, and garlic. Season with sage, thyme, and rosemary. Bring to a boil, reduce heat, and cook 1 hour.
2. Remove chicken from the pot, shred with a fork, and set aside.
3. Stir the sweet potato into the pot. Continue cooking about 5 minutes, until sweet potato is slightly tender. Mix in the zucchini, yellow squash, and escarole. Continue cooking 15 minutes.
4. Return the shredded chicken to the pot. Cook until heated through. Increase the amount of broth if the soup seems too thick.

SEASONED ROASTED ROOT VEGETABLES

Servings: 10 | Prep: 30m | Cooks: 45m | Total: 1h15m

NUTRITION FACTS

Calories: 149 | Carbohydrates: 29.9g | Fat: 3.1g | Protein: 3.4g | Cholesterol: 0mg

INGREDIENTS

- olive oil cooking spray
- 3 carrots, cut into large chunks

- 1 butternut squash - peeled, seeded, and cut into 1-inch pieces
- 1 large sweet potato, peeled and cut into 1-inch cubes
- 1 (10 ounce) package frozen Brussels sprouts, thawed and halved
- 1 onion, halved and thickly sliced
- 1 parsnip, peeled and sliced
- 2 tablespoons olive oil, or as needed
- 1 teaspoon ground thyme
- 1 teaspoon dried rosemary
- 1 pinch salt
- ground black pepper to taste

DIRECTIONS

1. Preheat oven to 400 degrees F (200 degrees C). Spray a baking sheet with cooking spray.
2. Combine butternut squash, sweet potato, Brussels sprouts, onion, parsnip, and carrots in a large bowl. Drizzle with olive oil and toss to coat. Add thyme, rosemary, salt, and black pepper; toss again. Transfer coated vegetables to the prepared baking sheet.
3. Roast vegetables in the preheated oven for 25 minutes; stir and continue roasting until vegetables are slightly brown and tender, about 20 more minutes.

WHAT THE ELLE...BAKED EGG ROLLS

Servings: 8 | Prep: 15m | Cooks: 20m | Total: 35m

NUTRITION FACTS

Calories: 150 | Carbohydrates: 16.9g | Fat: 3.6g | Protein: 12.4g | Cholesterol: 28mg

INGREDIENTS

- 2 cups grated carrots
- 1 (14.5 ounce) can bean sprouts, drained
- 1/2 cup chopped water chestnuts
- 1/4 cup chopped green bell pepper
- 1/4 cup chopped green onions
- 1 clove garlic, minced
- 2 cups finely diced cooked chicken
- 4 teaspoons cornstarch
- 1 tablespoon water
- 1 tablespoon light soy sauce
- 1 teaspoon vegetable oil
- 1 teaspoon brown sugar
- 1 pinch cayenne pepper
- 16 egg roll wrappers
- nonstick cooking spray

DIRECTIONS

1. Preheat oven to 425 degrees F (220 degrees C). Lightly grease a baking sheet.
2. Coat a large skillet with nonstick cooking spray and heat over medium heat; cook and stir carrots, bean sprouts, water chestnuts, green pepper, green onions, and garlic until vegetables are crisp, about 3 minutes. Stir in chicken until heated through, 3 to 5 minutes.
3. Combine cornstarch, water, soy sauce, 1 teaspoon oil, brown sugar, and cayenne in a small bowl; stir into chicken mixture. Bring to a boil over high heat and stir, cooking until sauce is thickened, about 2 minutes; remove from heat.
4. Spoon 1/4 cup chicken mixture on the bottom third of one egg roll wrapper. Fold sides toward center and roll tightly; place seam side down on prepared baking sheet. Repeat with remaining filling and wrappers. Spray top of egg rolls with nonstick cooking spray.
5. Bake in preheated oven until lightly browned, 10 to 15 minutes.

EASY BAKED APPLES

Servings: 6 | Prep: 5m | Cooks: 1h | Total: 1h5m

NUTRITION FACTS

Calories: 55 | Carbohydrates: 14.6g | Fat: 0.2g | Protein: 0.4g | Cholesterol: 0mg

INGREDIENTS

- 6 small apples, cored and halved
- 2 cups sugar-free diet orange-flavored carbonated beverage

DIRECTIONS

1. Preheat an oven to 350 degrees F (175 degrees C).
2. Arrange the apples into a baking dish with the cut sides facing down. Pour the orange beverage over the apples.
3. Bake in the preheated oven until the apples are tender, about 1 hour.

REFRESHING SWEET AND SPICY JICAMA SALAD (VEGAN)

Servings: 6 | Prep: 20m | Cooks: 30m | Total: 50m

NUTRITION FACTS

Calories: 119 | Carbohydrates: 28.3g | Fat: 0.5g | Protein: 3.3g | Cholesterol: 0mg

INGREDIENTS

- 1 large jicama, peeled and julienned
- 2 navel oranges, peeled and cut into chunks
- 1 large red bell pepper, cut into bite-size pieces
- 1/2 hothouse cucumber, diced
- 3 small sweet yellow peppers, sliced
- 2 small sweet orange peppers, sliced
- 4 radishes, thinly sliced
- 3 Thai chile peppers, minced
- 1/2 jalapeno pepper, diced
- 1/2 bunch cilantro, chopped
- 1 lemon, juiced
- ground black pepper to taste

DIRECTIONS

1. Combine jicama, orange chunks, red bell pepper, cucumber, sweet yellow and orange peppers, radishes, Thai chile peppers, jalapeno pepper, cilantro, lemon juice, and black pepper in a large bowl.
2. Cover the bowl with plastic wrap and refrigerate until flavors blend, about 30 minutes.

TUNA-STUFFED ZUCCHINI

Servings: 6 | Prep: 25m | Cooks: 25m | Total: 50m

NUTRITION FACTS

Calories: 193 | Carbohydrates: 18.2g | Fat: 4.7g | Protein: 19.4g | Cholesterol: 48mg

INGREDIENTS

- 3 zucchini, ends trimmed
- 4 (3 ounce) cans tuna, drained and flaked
- 1/4 onion, grated
- 1 tomato, finely chopped (optional)
- 1 cup dry bread crumbs
- 1 egg, beaten
- salt and ground black pepper to taste
- 1 tablespoon olive oil

DIRECTIONS

1. Fill a large pot with salted water, place the zucchini into the pot, and boil over medium heat for about 5 minutes to soften. Remove the zucchini, slice in half lengthwise, and allow to cool.
2. Preheat oven to 350 degrees F (175 degrees C). Lightly grease a 9x13-inch baking dish.

3. Scoop out the flesh from the zucchini halves, leaving a 1/2-inch shell. Set aside the scooped out flesh in a bowl.
4. Place the zucchini flesh into a bowl and mash well. Mix in the tuna, onion, tomato, bread crumbs, egg, salt, and black pepper. Lightly stuff the zucchini shells with the tuna mixture. Drizzle about 1/2 teaspoon of olive oil over each stuffed zucchini half.
5. Bake in the preheated oven until the tops are slightly browned, 20 to 25 minutes.

WARM APPLE CINNAMON COBBLER

Servings: 6 | Prep: 20m | Cooks: 30m | Total: 50m

NUTRITION FACTS

Calories: 258 | Carbohydrates: 42.2g | Fat: 10.1g | Protein: 2.9g | Cholesterol: 0mg

INGREDIENTS

- 4 apples - peeled, cored and sliced
- 1 cup water
- 2 teaspoons ground cinnamon
- 2 tablespoons cornstarch
- 1/4 cup fructose (fruit sugar)
- 1 cup whole wheat pastry flour
- 1 teaspoon baking powder
- 1/4 cup canola oil
- 1 tablespoon honey
- 1/2 cup lowfat buttermilk
- 1/2 cup lowfat buttermilk

DIRECTIONS

1. Preheat oven to 375 degrees F (190 degrees C).
2. In a large saucepan over medium heat, combine the apples, water, cinnamon, cornstarch and fructose. Cook until apples are soft and mixture is thickened, about 10 minutes.
3. Pour the apple mixture into a casserole dish.
4. Prepare biscuit dough by combining the whole-wheat pastry flour and baking powder. Add the oil and stir until well mixed. Add the honey and buttermilk; stir with a fork until flour mixture is moist. Add additional milk if necessary.
5. Drop biscuit dough by tablespoons on top of apples. Bake for 20 minutes or until biscuits are golden brown. Serve warm.

BLACK-EYED PEAS SPICY STYLE

Servings: 3 | Prep: 10m | Cooks: 30m | Total: 40m

NUTRITION FACTS

Calories: 119 | Carbohydrates: 21.4g | Fat: 0.8g | Protein: 7.1g | Cholesterol: 0mg

INGREDIENTS

- 1 (15.5 ounce) can black-eyed peas with liquid
- 1/2 onion, chopped
- minced jalapeno pepper to taste
- ground black pepper to taste

DIRECTIONS

1. In a medium-size pot, combine black-eyed peas, onion, jalapeno peppers, and black pepper (to taste). Heat all ingredients to simmer, let cook 30 minutes. Enjoy!.

SPICY DILL POTATO SALAD

Servings: 12 | Prep: 30m | Cooks: 35m | Total: 3h35m

NUTRITION FACTS

Calories: 153 | Carbohydrates: 25.8g | Fat: 3.9g | Protein: 5.5g | Cholesterol: 63mg

INGREDIENTS

- 3 pounds russet potatoes, peeled and cubed
- 4 eggs
- 2 red bell peppers
- 2 green bell peppers
- 1 red onion
- 2 cups reduced-fat mayonnaise
- 1/2 cup horseradish mustard
- 4 chipotle peppers in adobo sauce, chopped
- 1/4 cup adobo sauce from chipotle peppers
- 8 sprigs fresh dill, chopped
- 1 clove garlic, minced, or to taste
- 1 pinch ground cumin, or to taste
- salt and ground black pepper to taste

DIRECTIONS

1. Place the potatoes into a large pot and cover with salted water. Bring to a boil over high heat, then reduce heat to medium-low, cover, and simmer until tender, 10 to 15 minutes. Drain and allow to steam dry for a minute or two. Place the potatoes into a large bowl, and chill in the refrigerator until cold, about 1 hour.

2. While the potatoes are boiling, place the eggs into a saucepan in a single layer and fill with water to cover the eggs by 1 inch. Cover the saucepan and bring the water to a boil over high heat. Once the water is boiling, remove from the heat and let the eggs stand in the hot water for 15 minutes. Pour out the hot water, then cool the eggs under cold running water in the sink. Peel once cold. Chop the eggs, and place into the bowl with the potatoes.

3. Preheat oven to 425 degrees F (220 degrees C). Cut the bell peppers in half, and remove the seeds, core, and stems. Place the bell peppers onto a baking sheet, cut sides down. Cut the onion in half, and place it onto the baking sheet, cut sides down.

4. Roast the peppers and onion in the preheated oven until the skin of the vegetables has charred in places, about 25 minutes. Remove any large pieces of burned skin, and chop the peppers and onions. Transfer into the bowl with the potatoes and eggs.

5. In a bowl, stir together the mayonnaise, horseradish mustard, chipotle peppers, adobo sauce, dill, garlic, cumin, and salt and pepper until thoroughly combined. Pour the dressing over the potato mixture, and lightly toss until the potatoes, eggs, and vegetables are thoroughly coated with dressing. Chill before serving.

BENGALI DHAL

Servings: 4 | Prep: 15m | Cooks: 30m | Total: 45m

NUTRITION FACTS

Calories: 224 | Carbohydrates: 34.3g | Fat: 4.1g | Protein: 13.2g | Cholesterol: 0mg

INGREDIENTS

- 1 cup red lentils
- 3 cups water
- 1 cup onion, thinly sliced, divided
- 4 cloves garlic, coarsely chopped, divided
- 1/2 teaspoon ground turmeric
- 1 bay leaf
- 3/4 cup cherry tomatoes
- 1/2 teaspoon salt
- 2 (2 inch) whole serrano chile peppers (optional)
- 1 tablespoon vegetable oil
- 2 tablespoons chopped cilantro

DIRECTIONS

1. Wash the lentils in a strainer. Combine the lentils and water in a saucepan over medium-high heat. Add half of the sliced onions and garlic, reserving the rest for later. Stir in the turmeric, bay leaf, tomatoes, and salt. Add the chiles, leaving them whole to add flavor or cut in half to add heat. When

the mixture begins to boil, reduce the heat to a simmer. Cook until the lentils break apart and thicken slightly, about 20 minutes.

2. Meanwhile, in a skillet, heat the vegetable oil over medium heat until the oil shimmers. Add the reserved sliced onions; cook and stir until the onion has softened and turned translucent, about 5 minutes. Reduce heat to medium-low, and continue cooking and stirring until the onion is very tender and dark brown, 15 to 20 minutes more. Stir in the rest of the chopped garlic and cook, stirring constantly, until the garlic is fragrant and tender, about 2 minutes.

3. Pour the contents of the skillet into the cooked lentils and stir. Garnish with chopped cilantro.

FIESTA CHICKEN FROM UNCLE BEN'S®

Servings: 6 | Prep: 35m | Cooks: 35m | Total: 1h

NUTRITION FACTS

Calories: 94 | Carbohydrates: 16.1g | Fat: 2.8g | Protein: 3.2g | Cholesterol: 0mg

INGREDIENTS

- Nonstick cooking spray
- 3 cups water
- 1 1/2 tablespoons chili powder
- 1/4 cup chopped cilantro
- 3/4 cup salsa (mild)
- 3/4 cup red pepper, diced
- 1 cup chopped onion
- 3 cups UNCLE BEN'S® Fast & Natural™ Whole Grain Instant Brown Rice
- 6 chicken breast halves
- 1 cup corn kernels, frozen or canned

DIRECTIONS

1. Heat oil in a saute pan over medium heat. Add onion, and cook and stir for 3 minutes. Add tomatoes, zucchini, and green pepper. Stir. Season to taste with salt and black pepper. Reduce heat, cover, and simmer for 5 minutes.
2. Stir in rice and water. Cover, and cook over low heat for 20 minutes.

SUMMER FRUIT SALAD WITH A LEMON, HONEY, AND MINT DRESSING

Servings: 8 | Prep: 20m | Cooks: 1h | Total: 1h20m

NUTRITION FACTS

Calories: 99 | Carbohydrates: 24.8g | Fat: 0.5g | Protein: 1.5g | Cholesterol: 0mg

INGREDIENTS

- 4 cups cubed seeded watermelon
- 2 cups sliced fresh strawberries
- 2 large fresh peaches, cut into cubes
- 2 large nectarines, cut into cubes
- 1 red Anjou pear, cut into cubes
- 1 cup seedless grapes, halved
- 2 lemons, juiced
- 1/4 cup minced fresh mint (chocolate mint preferred)
- 1/2 lemon, zested
- 1 tablespoon honey (fireweed honey preferred)

DIRECTIONS

1. Combine watermelon, strawberries, peaches, nectarines, pear, and grapes in a large mixing bowl.
2. Whisk lemon juice, mint, lemon zest, and honey together in a small bowl; drizzle over the fruit mixture and toss to coat.
3. Refrigerate 1 hour before serving.

VANILLA GRANOLA

Servings: 16 | Prep: 10m | Cooks: 25m | Total: 35m

NUTRITION FACTS

Calories: 131 | Carbohydrates: 20g | Fat: 4.3g | Protein: 3.9g | Cholesterol: 0mg

INGREDIENTS

- non-stick cooking spray
- 4 cups rolled oats
- 1 cup sliced almonds
- 1/2 cup granular sucralose sweetener with brown sugar (such as Splenda® Brown Sugar Blend)
- 1/4 teaspoon salt
- 1/4 teaspoon ground cinnamon
- 1 cup applesauce
- 2 tablespoons white sugar
- 4 teaspoons vanilla extract

DIRECTIONS

1. Preheat oven to 300 degrees F (150 degrees C). Lightly spray large baking sheet with non-stick cooking spray.

2. Mix oats, almonds, sweetener, salt, and cinnamon in a large bowl.
3. Stir applesauce and sugar together in a small saucepan; bring to a simmer over medium heat and immediately remove from heat. Stir vanilla into the applesauce mixture; pour over the oats mixture and toss to coat. Spread the mixture onto the prepared baking dish.
4. Bake until golden brown, stirring occasionally, 20 to 30 minutes. Place baking sheet on a cooling rack until granola is completely cooled.

OVEN-FRIED BANANAS

Servings: 2 | Prep: 10m | Cooks: 10m | Total: 20m

NUTRITION FACTS

Calories: 119 | Carbohydrates: 25.6g | Fat: 1.4g | Protein: 2.6g | Cholesterol: 0mg

INGREDIENTS

- cooking spray
- 1/4 cup dry bread crumbs
- 1 tablespoon granular no-calorie sucralose sweetener (such as Splenda®)
- 1/4 teaspoon ground cinnamon
- 1/4 teaspoon ground ginger
- 1 pinch salt
- 1 large banana, cut into slices

DIRECTIONS

1. Preheat an oven to 425 degrees F (220 degrees C).
2. Line a baking sheet with parchment paper and spray with cooking spray.
3. Combine bread crumbs, no-calorie sweetener, cinnamon, ginger, and salt in a bowl.
4. Spray banana slices on both sides with the cooking spray.
5. Roll banana slices in the bread crumb mixture to coat, and arrange slices on the prepared baking sheet.
6. Lightly spray the banana slices again.
7. Bake in the preheated oven until crisp, 10 to 15 minutes.

SPICY BRUSSELS SPROUTS

Servings: 4 | Prep: 15m | Cooks: 30m | Total: 45m

NUTRITION FACTS

Calories: 64 | Carbohydrates: 13.4g | Fat: 0.4g | Protein: 4.1g | Cholesterol: 0mg

INGREDIENTS

- 1 pound Brussels sprouts
- 2 cloves garlic, thinly sliced
- 1/2 teaspoon cayenne pepper
- 1/2 teaspoon crushed red pepper flakes
- 2 green onions, chopped
- 2 tablespoons Dijon mustard
- 1 tablespoon lemon juice
- salt and ground black pepper to taste

DIRECTIONS

1. Place a steamer insert into a saucepan, and fill with water to just below the bottom of the steamer. Cover, and bring the water to a boil over high heat. Add the Brussels sprouts, and season with garlic, cayenne pepper, and red pepper flakes. Recover, and steam to your desired degree of tenderness, about 30 minutes for very tender.
2. Remove the Brussels sprouts from the steamer and place into a bowl. Add the green onions, mustard, and lemon juice. Season to taste with salt and pepper. Toss until evenly coated.

HONEY ORANGE GREEN BEANS

Servings: 4 | Prep: 15m | Cooks: 10m | Total: 45m

NUTRITION FACTS

Calories: 88 | Carbohydrates: 19.6g | Fat: 1.3g | Protein: 1.6g | Cholesterol: 0mg

INGREDIENTS

- 3 tablespoons honey
- 1/2 orange, zested
- 2 cloves garlic, minced
- 1 teaspoon soy sauce
- 1 1/2 teaspoons balsamic vinegar
- 1 dash ground black pepper
- 1 tablespoon water
- 2 cups fresh green beans, trimmed
- 1 teaspoon extra-virgin olive oil
- 1 tomato, diced

DIRECTIONS

1. Stir the honey, orange zest, garlic, soy sauce, balsamic vinegar, pepper, and water together in a bowl. Add the green beans and toss to coat. Allow to soak for 20 minutes, mixing every 5 minutes.
2. Heat the olive oil in a saucepan over low heat; add the green beans to the hot oil and cover the saucepan. Pour the green beans and sauce into the pan and cook, shaking the pan regularly, until the

beans are slightly tender, about 5 minutes. Add the tomatoes to the green beans, replace the cover, and continue cooking until the green beans are cooked though yet slightly crispy, about 5 minutes more.

SPICY CHIPOTLE BLACK-EYED PEAS

Servings: 20 | Prep: 20m | Cooks: 8h | Total: 8h20m

NUTRITION FACTS

Calories: 156 | Carbohydrates: 26.9g | Fat: 2.7g | Protein: 9.2g | Cholesterol: 0mg

INGREDIENTS

- 2 tablespoons olive oil
- 1 tablespoon balsamic vinegar
- 1 cup chopped orange bell pepper
- 1 cup chopped celery
- 1 cup chopped carrot
- 1 cup chopped onion
- 1 teaspoon minced garlic
- 2 (16 ounce) packages dry black-eyed peas
- 4 cups water
- 4 teaspoons vegetable bouillon base (such as Better Than Bouillon® Vegetable Base)
- 1 (7 ounce) can chipotle peppers in adobo sauce, chopped, sauce reserved
- 2 teaspoons liquid mesquite smoke flavoring
- 2 teaspoons ground cumin
- 1/2 teaspoon ground black pepper

DIRECTIONS

1. Heat the olive oil and balsamic vinegar in a skillet; cook and stir the orange bell pepper, celery, carrot, onion, and garlic in the hot oil until the onion is translucent, 5 to 8 minutes. Transfer the mixture to a slow cooker; mix in the black-eyed peas, water, and vegetable base, stirring to dissolve the vegetable base. Stir in the chipotle peppers, about 1 tablespoon of the reserved adobo sauce (or to taste), liquid smoke, cumin, and black pepper.
2. Cook in the slow cooker on Low until the black-eyed peas are very tender and the flavors are blended, about 8 hours.

BEER SIMMERED BEANS

Servings: 6 | Prep: 10m | Cooks: 10m | Total: 20m

NUTRITION FACTS

Calories: 119 | Carbohydrates: 19.9g | Fat: 0.8g | Protein: 6.5g | Cholesterol: 0mg

INGREDIENTS

- 1 (15 ounce) can pinto beans, rinsed and drained
- 1 (15 ounce) can kidney beans, rinsed and drained
- 1 cup light beer
- 2 jalapeno peppers, minced
- 2 cloves garlic, minced
- 1 1/2 teaspoons cumin
- 1/4 teaspoon salt

DIRECTIONS

1. Combine pinto beans, kidney beans, beer, jalapenos, garlic, cumin, and salt in a large saucepan. Simmer for 10 minutes. Serve warm or chilled.

GRILLED CHICKEN CITRUS SALAD

Servings: 4 | Prep: 30m | Cooks: 15m | Total: 2h45m | Additional: 2h

NUTRITION FACTS

Calories: 238 | Carbohydrates: 26.1g | Fat: 2.2g | Protein: 30g | Cholesterol: 66mg

INGREDIENTS

- 1/2 cup orange juice
- 1/4 cup lime juice
- 2 shallots, minced
- 2 cloves garlic, minced
- 1 teaspoon chili powder
- 1 teaspoon ground cumin
- 1 teaspoon white sugar
- 4 (4 ounce) skinless, boneless chicken breast halves
- 8 cups torn romaine lettuce
- 2 oranges - peeled, segmented, and chopped
- 2 stalks celery, sliced
- 4 green onions, chopped

DIRECTIONS

1. In a mixing bowl, whisk together orange juice, lime juice, shallots, garlic, chili powder, cumin, and sugar. Pour 1/2 of this mixture into a large, resealable plastic bag, and add the chicken breasts. Seal, and refrigerate for at least 2 hours. Refrigerate the remaining dressing.

2. Preheat an outdoor grill for medium-high heat. In a large salad bowl, toss romaine lettuce with oranges, celery, and green onions. Set aside.
3. Lightly oil grate, and place chicken on grill. Discard the marinade from the chicken. Cook for 6 to 8 minutes each side, or until juices run clear when pierced with a fork. Remove chicken from grill, and slice into thin strips.
4. Toss salad with reserved dressing, and top with sliced chicken.

BOILED MUSTARD POTATOES
Servings: 6 | Prep: 15m | Cooks: 25m | Total: 40m

NUTRITION FACTS

Calories: 135 | Carbohydrates: 28.7g | Fat: 1g | Protein: 4.1g | Cholesterol: 0mg

INGREDIENTS

- 6 cups water
- 1/2 teaspoon salt, or to taste
- 1/2 cup prepared yellow mustard, or to taste
- 5 large Yukon Gold potatoes, peeled and halved

DIRECTIONS

1. Whisk the water, yellow mustard, and salt together in a large saucepan. Bring to a boil over medium heat, and stir in the potatoes. Reduce heat to medium-low, and simmer until tender, 25 to 30 minutes. Drain liquid, and serve.

A NEW GREEN BEAN CASSEROLE
Servings: 6 | Prep: 20m | Cooks: 1h | Total: 1h20m

NUTRITION FACTS

Calories: 97 | Carbohydrates: 19.5g | Fat: 1.3g | Protein: 4.6g | Cholesterol: 2mg

INGREDIENTS

- 1 1/2 pounds fresh green beans, trimmed
- 4 cups sliced onions
- 2 tablespoons balsamic vinegar, or more if needed
- 3 cloves garlic, chopped
- 2 teaspoons white sugar
- 1 teaspoon dried basil
- 1 teaspoon dried oregano
- 1/4 cup shredded Parmesan cheese, or to taste
- halved grape tomatoes

DIRECTIONS

1. Bring a large pot of lightly salted water to a boil; cook green beans at a boil until tender yet firm to the bite, 5 to 10 minutes; drain and transfer to a 9x13-inch dish.
2. Cook and stir onions, vinegar, garlic, sugar, basil, and oregano in a skillet over medium heat until onions are softened and translucent, about 5 minutes. Reduce heat to medium-low, and continue cooking and stirring until onions are very tender and dark brown, 15 to 20 minutes more.
3. Preheat oven to 400 degrees F (200 degrees C).
4. Spread onion mixture over green beans and top with Parmesan cheese. Arrange tomatoes, cut sides down, atop Parmesan cheese layer.
5. Bake in the preheated oven until cheese is melted and bubbling, about 35 minutes.

ZUCCHINI-TOMATO SAUTE

Servings: 1 | Prep: 5m | Cooks: 8h | Total: 8h5m

NUTRITION FACTS

Calories: 203 | Carbohydrates: 33.3g | Fat: 5g | Protein: 8.1g | Cholesterol: 0mg

INGREDIENTS

- 1/2 cup almond milk
- 1/4 cup fresh raspberries
- 1/4 cup rolled oats
- 2 tablespoons powdered peanut butter (such as PB2®)
- 1 1/2 teaspoons chia seeds
- 1 teaspoon white sugar

DIRECTIONS

1. Mix almond milk, raspberries, rolled oats, powdered peanut butter, chia seeds, and sugar together in a container. Cover and refrigerate until oats are soft, 8 hours to overnight.

CURRIED CREAM OF ANY VEGGIE SOUP

Servings: 6 | Prep: 15m | Cooks: 30m | Total: 45m

NUTRITION FACTS

Calories: 139 | Carbohydrates: 23.2g | Fat: 3.1g | Protein: 7g | Cholesterol: 2mg

INGREDIENTS

- 1 tablespoon vegetable oil
- 4 cups chopped mixed vegetables

- 1 onion, chopped
- 1 clove garlic, minced
- 1 tablespoon curry powder
- 4 cups chicken broth
- 2 tablespoons all-purpose flour
- 2 cups nonfat milk
- salt and pepper to taste

DIRECTIONS

1. Heat oil in a large saucepan over medium heat. Saute onion and garlic until tender. Stir in curry, and cook for 2 minutes, stirring constantly. Add broth and vegetables, and bring to a boil. Simmer 20 minutes, or until tender.
2. Dissolve flour in milk, then stir into the soup. Simmer until thickened. Season with salt and pepper.

COLORFUL BULGUR SALAD

Servings: 4 | Prep: 15m | Cooks: 10m | Total: 3h20m

NUTRITION FACTS

Calories: 65 | Carbohydrates: 13.8g | Fat: 0.7g | Protein: 2.9g | Cholesterol: 0mg

INGREDIENTS

- 1/2 cup cracked bulgur wheat
- 1/2 cup chicken broth
- 1 small cucumber, seeded and chopped
- 1 tomato, chopped
- 1 carrot, shredded
- 3 green onions, thinly sliced
- 3 tablespoons fresh lime juice
- 3/4 tablespoon chili powder
- 1 pinch garlic powder

DIRECTIONS

1. Place bulgur in a colander and rinse under cold running water. Drain and transfer to a small bowl.
2. In a small saucepan bring the chicken broth to a boil. Stir in the bulgur, remove from the heat and let stand for 1 hour.
3. Stir in the cucumbers, tomatoes, carrots, and green onions into the bulgur.
4. In a small bowl whisk the lime juice, chili powder and garlic powder together. Pour over the bulgur mixture and stir until combined. Cover and chill for 2 hours before serving. Stir before serving.

REDUCED FAT FRENCH TOAST

Servings: 6 | Prep: 5m | Cooks: 10m | Total: 15m

NUTRITION FACTS

Calories: 77 | Carbohydrates: 11.9g | Fat: 1.3g | Protein: 5.4g | Cholesterol: <1mg

INGREDIENTS

- 1/2 cup egg substitute
- 2/3 cup skim milk
- 1 teaspoon vanilla extract
- 1/2 teaspoon ground cinnamon
- 6 slices reduced calorie white bread

DIRECTIONS

1. Beat together egg substitute, milk, vanilla and cinnamon. Dip bread slices in egg mixture until both sides are soaked.
2. Spray a skillet or frying pan with cooking spray and heat over medium high heat. Place bread slices into pan and cook until golden brown on both sides .

OVEN BAKED VEGETABLES

Servings: 6 | Prep: 10m | Cooks: 25m | Total: 35m

NUTRITION FACTS

Calories: 98 | Carbohydrates: 22.5g | Fat: 0.2g | Protein: 2.1g | Cholesterol: 0mg

INGREDIENTS

- 1 vegetable cooking spray
- 2 potatoes, cubed
- 1 carrot, sliced
- 2 onions, sliced
- 1 green bell pepper, chopped
- 1/3 cup fat free Italian-style dressing
- 1/8 teaspoon garlic salt
- 1/4 teaspoon cayenne pepper
- 1/8 teaspoon onion salt

DIRECTIONS

1. Preheat oven to 350 degrees F (175 degrees C). Spray a 9 x 13 inch baking pan with cooking spray.
2. In prepared pan combine potatoes, carrots, onions and bell pepper.
3. In a small bowl combine Italian dressing, garlic salt, cayenne pepper and onion salt. Pour over vegetables.
4. Bake, covered, for 15 minutes. Uncover, stir and bake for 10 minutes more.

CARIBBEAN SLAW

Servings: 8 | Prep: 20m | Cooks: 1h | Total: 1h20m

NUTRITION FACTS

Calories: 61 | Carbohydrates: 13.1g | Fat: 0.6g | Protein: 2.1g | Cholesterol: <1mg

INGREDIENTS

- 1/2 head green cabbage, shredded
- 1 red bell pepper, thinly sliced
- 1/2 red onion, thinly sliced
- 2 carrots, peeled and shredded
- 1 mango - peeled, seeded, and diced
- 1/2 cup fresh cilantro, chopped
- 1/3 cup nonfat plain yogurt
- 2 tablespoons reduced-fat mayonnaise
- 1 tablespoon prepared yellow mustard
- 1 tablespoon apple cider vinegar
- 1 teaspoon agave nectar
- salt and black pepper to taste
- 1 dash habanero hot sauce, or more to taste

DIRECTIONS

1. Toss the cabbage, red bell pepper, red onion, carrots, mango, and cilantro together in a large bowl.
2. Whisk the yogurt, mayonnaise, mustard, cider vinegar, agave nectar, salt, pepper, and hot sauce together in a small bowl; pour over the cabbage mixture and toss to coat. Allow the slaw to marinate in the refrigerator for at least 1 hour to allow the flavors to combine.

AIR FRYER GARLIC AND PARSLEY BABY POTATOES

Servings: 5 | Prep: 5m | Cooks: 20m | Total: 25m

NUTRITION FACTS

Calories: 89 | Carbohydrates: 20.1g | Fat: 0.1g | Protein: 2.4g | Cholesterol: 0mg

INGREDIENTS

- 1 pound baby potatoes, cut into quarters
- 1 tablespoon avocado oil
- 1/4 teaspoon salt
- 1/2 teaspoon granulated garlic
- 1/2 teaspoon dried parsley

DIRECTIONS

1. Preheat an air fryer to 350 degrees F (175 degrees C).
2. Combine potatoes and oil in a bowl and toss to coat. Add 1/4 teaspoon granulated garlic and 1/4 teaspoon parsley and toss to coat. Repeat with remaining garlic and parsley. Pour potatoes into the air fryer basket.
3. Place the basket in the air fryer and cook, tossing occasionally, until golden brown, about 20 to 25 minutes.

APPLE AND PUMPKIN DESSERT

Servings: 1 | Prep: 5m | Cooks: 4m | Total: 9m

NUTRITION FACTS

Calories: 88 | Carbohydrates: 23.8g | Fat: 0.4g | Protein: 1.2g | Cholesterol: 0mg

INGREDIENTS

- 2 (1 gram) packets sugar substitute
- 1 teaspoon pumpkin pie spice
- 1 Granny Smith apple - peeled, cored and chopped
- 1/4 cup canned pumpkin
- 2 tablespoons water

DIRECTIONS

1. Sprinkle 1/3 packet of sugar substitute and 1/3 teaspoon pumpkin pie spice in the bottom of a microwave-safe bowl. Layer 1/4 of the apple pieces into the bowl; repeat. Spread the pumpkin over the apples. Sprinkle the remaining sugar substitute and pumpkin pie spice on the pumpkin. Top with the remaining apples. Pour the water over the mixture.
2. Cook in microwave on high for 3 1/2 minutes, stirring every minute.

FRUITY TUNA SALAD

Servings: 6 | Prep: 10m | Cooks: 1h | Total: 1h10m

NUTRITION FACTS

Calories: 159 | Carbohydrates: 27.2g | Fat: 0.8g | Protein: 12.6g | Cholesterol: 14mg

INGREDIENTS

- 2 (5 ounce) cans tuna, drained
- 1 cup chopped dates
- 1 1/2 cups chopped celery
- 1 large apple - peeled, cored and diced
- 1/2 cup lemon yogurt
- 1 tablespoon minced onion
- 2 teaspoons lemon juice
- 1 teaspoon ground curry powder

DIRECTIONS

1. In a large bowl, mix the tuna, dates, celery and apple.
2. In a separate bowl, whisk together the yogurt, onion, lemon juice, and curry powder. Pour over tuna mixture and gently toss to coat. Refrigerate 1 hour, or until chilled.

INSTANT POT® APPLE PIE STEEL CUT OATS

Servings: 4 | Prep: 5m | Cooks: 15m | Total: 30m

NUTRITION FACTS

Calories: 171 | Carbohydrates: 32.6g | Fat: 2.6g | Protein: 5.1g | Cholesterol: 0mg

INGREDIENTS

- 3 cups water
- 1 cup steel-cut oats
- 1 apple, or more to taste, chopped
- 1 1/2 teaspoons ground cinnamon
- 1/2 teaspoon salt
- 1/4 teaspoon ground nutmeg

DIRECTIONS

1. Combine water, oats, apple, cinnamon, salt, and nutmeg in a multi-functional pressure cooker (such as Instant Pot(R)). Close and lock the lid. Seal vent. Select Manual function; set timer for 5 minutes. Allow 10 to 15 minutes for pressure to build.

2. Release pressure using the natural-release method according to manufacturer's instructions, about 10 minutes. Release remaining pressure naturally. Stir and remove pot carefully with oven mitts.

EASY SOUTHERN FRIED GREEN TOMATOES

Servings: 8 | Prep: 15m | Cooks: 10m | Total: 25m

NUTRITION FACTS

Calories: 189 | Carbohydrates: 31.5g | Fat: 4.7g | Protein: 5.8g | Cholesterol: 46mg

INGREDIENTS

- waxed paper
- 2 large eggs
- 2 tablespoons water
- 1 cup all-purpose flour
- 1 cup yellow cornmeal
- sea salt to taste
- freshly ground black pepper to taste
- 2 pounds green tomatoes, sliced
- 1 cup canola oil for frying, or as needed

DIRECTIONS

1. Line a baking sheet with waxed paper.
2. Beat eggs and water in a shallow bowl. Place flour and cornmeal in 2 separate shallow bowls. Season cornmeal with salt and pepper.
3. Dip each tomato slice into flour, then dip into egg mixture. Press tomato into cornmeal mixture, shaking off excess. Transfer tomato to prepared baking sheet. Repeat with remaining tomato slices, arranging tomatoes in a single layer.
4. Heat about 1/4 inch canola oil in a large skillet over medium heat until oil begins to shimmer. Fry tomatoes in batches until golden and crisp, 3 to 4 minutes per side. Drain on paper towel-lined plates. Repeat with remaining tomatoes.

PROTEIN-PACKED SPICY VEGAN QUINOA WITH EDAMAME

Servings: 8 | Prep: 15m | Cooks: 30m | Total: 45m

NUTRITION FACTS

Calories: 94 | Carbohydrates: 16.1g | Fat: 2.8g | Protein: 3.2g | Cholesterol: 0mg

INGREDIENTS

- 3 1/2 cups water
- 2 cups quinoa, rinsed
- 4 teaspoons vegetable bouillon (such as Better Than Bouillon®)
- 2 1/2 cups frozen shelled edamame (green soybeans)
- 1 tablespoon olive oil
- 2 sweet onions, chopped

- 2 bell peppers, chopped
- 2 tablespoons minced fresh ginger
- 6 cloves garlic, minced
- 1/4 cup reduced-sodium soy sauce
- 2 tablespoons chopped fresh cilantro
- 1 tablespoon hot chile paste (such as sambal oelek), or to taste (optional)

DIRECTIONS

1. Bring water, quinoa, and vegetable bouillon to a boil in a large pot; stir in edamame, cover, and simmer until quinoa is tender, 15 to 20 minutes.
2. Heat olive oil in a large skillet over medium heat; cook and stir onions and bell peppers until onions are translucent, about 5 minutes. Add ginger and garlic; cook and stir until fragrant, about 2 minutes. Remove from heat; stir in soy sauce, cilantro, and chile paste.
3. Stir onion mixture into quinoa mixture; simmer, stirring occasionally, until excess broth has been absorbed, about 5 minutes.

PROTEIN-PACKED SPICY VEGAN QUINOA WITH EDAMAME

Servings: 8 | Prep: 15m | Cooks: 30m | Total: 45m

NUTRITION FACTS

Calories: 206 | Carbohydrates: 34.9g | Fat: 4.6g | Protein: 7.3g | Cholesterol: 0mg

INGREDIENTS

- 3 1/2 cups water
- 2 cups quinoa, rinsed
- 4 teaspoons vegetable bouillon (such as Better Than Bouillon®)
- 2 1/2 cups frozen shelled edamame (green soybeans)

- 2 bell peppers, chopped
- 2 tablespoons minced fresh ginger
- 6 cloves garlic, minced
- 1/4 cup reduced-sodium soy sauce

- 1 tablespoon olive oil
- 2 sweet onions, chopped
- 2 tablespoons chopped fresh cilantro
- 1 tablespoon hot chile paste (such as sambal oelek), or to taste (optional)

DIRECTIONS

1. Bring water, quinoa, and vegetable bouillon to a boil in a large pot; stir in edamame, cover, and simmer until quinoa is tender, 15 to 20 minutes.
2. Heat olive oil in a large skillet over medium heat; cook and stir onions and bell peppers until onions are translucent, about 5 minutes. Add ginger and garlic; cook and stir until fragrant, about 2 minutes. Remove from heat; stir in soy sauce, cilantro, and chile paste.
3. Stir onion mixture into quinoa mixture; simmer, stirring occasionally, until excess broth has been absorbed, about 5 minutes.

CALICO SLAW

Servings: 8 | Prep: 20m | Cooks: 30m | Total: 50m

NUTRITION FACTS

Calories: 81 | Carbohydrates: 19.4g | Fat: 0.3g | Protein: 2.2g | Cholesterol: 0mg

INGREDIENTS

- 1 medium head green cabbage, shredded
- 3 carrots, shredded
- 1 green bell pepper, seeded and thinly sliced
- 1 red bell pepper, seeded and thinly sliced
- 1 yellow bell pepper, seeded and thinly sliced
- 1 Red Delicious apple, cored and chopped
- 1 Golden Delicious apple, cored and chopped
- 2 tablespoons apple cider vinegar
- 2 tablespoons white sugar
- 1/2 teaspoon fine sea salt
- ground black pepper, to taste

DIRECTIONS

1. Toss the cabbage, carrots, green bell pepper, red bell pepper, Red Delicious apple, and Golden Delicious apple together in a large bowl.
2. Whisk the apple cider vinegar, sugar, and sea salt together in a small bowl; season with black pepper. Pour the vinegar mixture over the cabbage mixture and gently toss to coat. Cover the bowl with plastic wrap and refrigerate at least 30 minutes.

BANANA CHIA PUDDING

Servings: 6 | Prep: 10m | Cooks: 2h | Total: 2h10m

NUTRITION FACTS

Calories: 112 | Carbohydrates: 20.5g | Fat: 3.4g | Protein: 1.6g | Cholesterol: 0mg

INGREDIENTS

- 1 1/2 cups vanilla-flavored flax milk
- 1 large banana, cut in chunks
- 7 tablespoons chia seeds
- 3 tablespoons honey
- 1 teaspoon vanilla extract
- 1/8 teaspoon sea salt

DIRECTIONS

1. Put milk, banana, chia seeds, honey, vanilla extract, and sea salt in respective order in the blender; blend until smooth. Pour mixture into a bowl and refrigerate until thickened, at least 2 hours. Spoon mixture into small bowls to serve.

DUCK FAT-ROASTED BRUSSELS SPROUTS

Servings: 4 | Prep: 20m | Cooks: 15m | Total: 35m

NUTRITION FACTS

Calories: 125 | Carbohydrates: 23.4g | Fat: 3.1g | Protein: 8g | Cholesterol: 2mg

INGREDIENTS

- 2 tablespoons duck fat, or more as needed
- 2 pounds Brussels sprouts, trimmed and halved lengthwise
- salt and freshly ground black pepper to taste
- 1 pinch cayenne pepper, or more to taste
- 1 lemon, juiced

DIRECTIONS

1. Preheat an oven to 450 degrees F (230 degrees C). Line a baking sheet with parchment paper or a silicone baking mat.
2. Heat duck fat in a small saucepan until melted.

3. Combine Brussels sprouts, salt, black pepper, cayenne pepper, and melted duck fat in a large bowl until Brussels sprouts are evenly coated. Transfer to the prepared baking sheet.
4. Bake in the preheated oven until Brussels sprouts are browned and tender, but still slightly firm, 15 to 20 minutes. Flip Brussels sprouts over halfway through. Top with freshly squeezed lemon juice.

INSTANT POT® STEAMED ARTICHOKES

Servings: 4 | Prep: 5m | Cooks: 20m | Total: 30m

NUTRITION FACTS

Calories: 64 | Carbohydrates: 14.6g | Fat: 0.2g | Protein: 4.3g | Cholesterol: 0mg

INGREDIENTS

- 1 cup water
- 2 cloves garlic
- 1 bay leaf
- 1/2 teaspoon salt
- 4 artichokes, trimmed and stemmed
- 2 tablespoons lemon juice

DIRECTIONS

1. Combine water, garlic, bay leaf, and salt inside a multi-functional pressure cooker (such as Instant Pot(R)). Place steamer in the pot. Add artichokes, trimmed top facing up; drizzle with lemon juice. Close and lock the lid. Select high pressure according to manufacturer's instructions; set timer for 10 minutes. Allow 10 to 15 minutes for pressure to build.
2. Release pressure carefully using the quick-release method according to manufacturer's instructions, about 5 minutes. Unlock and remove lid.
3. Cool until easily handled. Pull off outer petals one at a time. Pull through teeth to remove the soft portion of the petal. Discard remaining petal. Spoon out fuzzy center near the stem and discard. Eat the bottom whole or cut into pieces.

VEGGIE-PACKED MEATLOAF WITH QUINOA

Servings: 8 | Prep: 20m | Cooks: 55m | Total: 1h20m

NUTRITION FACTS

Calories: 232 | Carbohydrates: 22.9g | Fat: 2.8g | Protein: 27.8g | Cholesterol: 82mg

INGREDIENTS

- 1 onion, quartered
- 4 cloves garlic, peeled
- 1 1/2 pounds lean ground meat (turkey or chicken)
- 1 1/4 cups quinoa, cooked then cooled

- 1 large carrot, quartered
- 1 celery stalk, quartered
- 2 1/2 cups baby spinach
- 1 egg, lightly beaten
- 3 tablespoons low-sodium soy sauce
- 1/2 teaspoon ground black pepper
- 1/4 cup ketchup or barbecue sauce

DIRECTIONS

1. Preheat the oven to 425 degrees F and line a small baking sheet with parchment paper.
2. Place onion and garlic in a food processor and pulse until finely chopped. Transfer to a large skillet. Add carrot and celery to the food processor, and pulse until chopped. Add spinach and pulse a few times more. Add to the skillet. Place the skillet over medium heat and cook, stirring until vegetables release liquid. Continue cooking until liquid evaporates and vegetables begin to brown, about 8 minutes; add water a tablespoon at a time, if necessary, to keep vegetables from sticking. Transfer to a large bowl.
3. Add egg, ground meat, quinoa, soy sauce and black pepper to the bowl, and mix gently with your hands. Scrape mixture onto the baking sheet and form into a loaf approximately 4 inches wide and 10 inches long; wet your hands if the mixture is very sticky. Spread top of loaf with ketchup or barbecue sauce. Bake until cooked through and browned, about 40 minutes. Cool 5 minutes before slicing.

BONE BROTH

Servings: 8 | Prep: 10m | Cooks: 1d30m | Total: 1d40m

NUTRITION FACTS

Calories: 49 | Carbohydrates: 11.4g | Fat: 0.2g | Protein: 1.8g | Cholesterol: 0mg

INGREDIENTS

- cooking spray
- 1 (6 ounce) can tomato paste
- 2 pounds beef bones
- 6 cups cool water, or as needed
- 2 onions, thickly sliced
- 2 carrots
- 3 cloves garlic, crushed
- 2 bay leaves

DIRECTIONS

1. Preheat oven to 400 degrees F (200 degrees C). Spray a roasting pan with cooking spray.
2. Spread tomato paste onto beef bones and place in the prepared roasting pan.

3. Bake in the preheated oven until bones begin to brown, about 30 minutes.
4. Transfer bones to a slow cooker and pour in enough water to cover bones. Add onions, carrots, garlic, and bay leaves to broth mixture.
5. Cook on Low for at least 24 hours.
6. Strain broth through a fine-mesh strainer into a container and refrigerate.

"SKINNY" CHICKEN TACOS

Servings: 4 | Prep: 15m | Cooks: 10m | Total: 35m | Additional: 10m

NUTRITION FACTS

Calories: 272 | Carbohydrates: 37.2g | Fat: 3.9g | Protein: 29.3g | Cholesterol: 65mg

INGREDIENTS

- 1 pound thinly sliced chicken breasts, cut into thin strips
- 3 limes, juiced, divided
- 2 teaspoons ground cumin, divided
- 2 teaspoons garlic powder, divided
- 2 teaspoons ground chipotle pepper, divided
- 2 red bell peppers, cut into thin strips
- 1 red onion, thinly sliced
- 2 jalapeno peppers - stemmed, seeded, and thinly sliced
- 4 multi-grain tortillas, or more to taste
- 1 bunch cilantro, chopped

DIRECTIONS

1. Combine chicken, juice of 1 lime, 1 teaspoon cumin, 1 teaspoon garlic powder, and 1 teaspoon chipotle pepper in a bowl; allow to marinate for 10 minutes.
2. Saute red bell peppers, onion, jalapeno peppers, juice of 1 lime, 1 teaspoon cumin, 1 teaspoon garlic powder, and 1 teaspoon chipotle pepper in a large non-stick skillet over medium-high heat until vegetables are tender yet crisp, about 5 minutes.
3. Transfer chicken mixture to a separate non-stick skillet over medium-high heat; saute until chicken is no longer pink in the center, 5 to 10 minutes.
4. Layer tortillas between paper towels on a microwave-safe plate; heat in microwave until warmed, 10 to 20 seconds.
5. Spoon vegetables and chicken onto tortillas; top with cilantro and lime juice.

TANGY JICAMA SLAW

Servings: 6 | Prep: 15m | Cooks: 10m | Total: 25m

NUTRITION FACTS

Calories: 67 | Carbohydrates: 16.6g | Fat: 0.2g | Protein: 1.3g | Cholesterol: 0mg

INGREDIENTS

- 1 jicama, peeled and chopped
- 1/4 cup fresh cilantro leaves, minced
- 1 large lime, juiced
- 1 lemon, juiced
- 1 (11 ounce) can mandarin orange segments, drained, liquid reserved
- salt to taste

DIRECTIONS

1. Combine the jicama, cilantro, lime juice, lemon juice, and mandarin orange segments with a small amount of the syrup from the can in a bowl; mix to evenly coat. Allow mixture to sit 10 minutes. Season with salt and stir just before serving.

KIWI SALSA

Servings: 6 | Prep: 15m | Cooks: 1h | Total: 1h15m

NUTRITION FACTS

Calories: 78 | Carbohydrates: 14g | Fat: 2.7g | Protein: 1.1g | Cholesterol: 0mg

INGREDIENTS

- 6 kiwis, peeled and diced
- 1 small onion, diced
- 1 jalapeno pepper, diced
- 2 tablespoons lime juice
- 1 tablespoon olive oil
- 1 teaspoon honey
- 1/2 teaspoon cumin
- 1/2 teaspoon curry powder

DIRECTIONS

1. Mix kiwi, onion, jalapeno pepper, lime juice, olive oil, honey, cumin, and curry powder together in bowl. Cover and allow to rest for 1 hour at room temperature. Refrigerate until ready to serve.

POLLO CON NOPALES (CHICKEN AND CACTUS)

Servings: 2 | Prep: 10m | Cooks: 20m | Total: 30m

NUTRITION FACTS

Calories: 174 | Carbohydrates: 11.9g | Fat: 3.2g | Protein: 25.7g | Cholesterol: 59mg

INGREDIENTS

- 2 skinless, boneless chicken breast halves
- 3 fresh tomatillos, husks removed
- 3 fresh jalapeno peppers, seeded
- 1 (16 ounce) jar canned nopales (cactus), drained

DIRECTIONS

1. Fill a pot with water and bring to a boil. Cook the chicken breasts in the boiling water until no longer pink in the center and the juices run clear, about 10 minutes. An instant-read thermometer inserted into the center should read at least 165 degrees F (74 degrees C). Drain and set aside to cool. Once cool, shred the chicken into small strands.
2. Fill the pot again with water and bring to a boil. Cook the tomatillos, jalapeno peppers, and nopales in the boiling water until the vegetables are all tender, about 5 minutes. Drain.
3. Blend the tomatillos and jalapeno peppers in a blender until smooth; pour into the pot with the shredded chicken and place over medium heat. Cut the nopales into small dice and add to the mixture. Allow the mixture to simmer until completely reheated, about 5 minutes.

MEXICAN MANGO

Servings: 2 | Prep: 5m | Cooks: 10m | Total: 15m

NUTRITION FACTS

Calories: 85 | Carbohydrates: 21.7g | Fat: 0.9g | Protein: 1.1g | Cholesterol: 0mg

INGREDIENTS

- 1/4 cup water
- 1 tablespoon chili powder
- 1 pinch salt
- 3 tablespoons lemon juice
- 1 mango - peeled, seeded, and sliced

DIRECTIONS

1. Bring water to a boil in a small saucepan. Stir in chili powder, salt, and lemon juice until smooth and hot. Add sliced mango and toss to coat; allow to soak up the chili sauce for a few minutes before serving.

www.ingramcontent.com/pod-product-compliance
Lightning Source LLC
Chambersburg PA
CBHW081939160726
47999CB00008B/2450